Unlearn pain

Jutta Richter

Unlearn pain

The Successful Techniques and Exercises of Psychological Pain Management

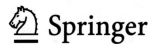 Springer

Jutta Richter
Psychologische Schmerztherapie
Bochum, Germany

ISBN 978-3-662-65701-0   ISBN 978-3-662-65702-7 (eBook)
https://doi.org/10.1007/978-3-662-65702-7

This Springer imprint is published by the registered company Springer-Verlag GmbH, DE, part of Springer Nature.
The registered company address is: Heidelberger Platz 3, 14197 Berlin, Germany

Preface to the 4th Edition

The growing number of people affected by pain testifies to the topicality and importance of pain and its chronification. Pain can have a major impact on a person's quality of life. Many sufferers with persistent pain seek alternatives and supplements to painkillers and medical therapies. What is required is self-help—practical everyday exercises that are available at any time and are also promising.

This legitimate concern affects many people who suffer from pain, regardless of its original cause. Pain can occur, for example, as a result of accidents, signs of wear and tear or in the so-called functional complaints. And sometimes they simply cannot—or no longer—be adequately explained.

This book is therefore written for people as follows:

- who have prolonged pain or whose pain is already called chronic
- who have acute pain and would like to be able to cope with it better
- who have already experienced a lot of pain in the past and would like to minimise expected pain (e.g. after operations)
- who have exhausted the exclusive medical possibilities, but whose pain reduction is not quite successful
- who want to treat their pain holistically, taking into account the psychological consequences of permanent pain: as a complement to painkillers, medical therapies and physiotherapy, or as a "gentle" alternative, with few side effects
- who are waiting for a psychologically oriented pain therapy and want to prepare this time sensibly—or to accompany an ongoing or carried out therapy
- who want to show initiative and take personal responsibility

This book is intended as a self-help guide for people suffering from pain. Of course, it does not replace medical and/or psychological care, but it can be a useful supplement to it. It is intended as a guide to learning and applying psychological techniques by means of practical exercises. In addition, information is given about psychosocial contexts and the development of chronic pain.

The intention of this book is to help those affected to better process, manage and reduce pain. Areas of life that could no longer be actively lived should be resumed and shaped—in short, the quality of life should be restored. The fact that psychological interventions are helpful and effective in this process is repeatedly shown by current psychological and interdisciplinary research results.

The demand and comments on the first three editions testify not only the great interest of patients, but also that of other professional groups, such as physicians psychotherapists and physiotherapists, who work with pain patients and are looking for psychologically oriented exercises to complement their own therapy.

Jutta Richter
Bochum, Germany
September 2020

Acknowledgements

My thanks to my husband and my children—for their patience, love and many ideas.

I would like to thank Professor Werner Siebert for his good wishes, Peter Otto for his successful drawing support, Dr. H. Schoeler for her support as a lector, Dr. A. Krätz from Springer-Verlag for her always friendly and competent advice, friends for their inspiration—and all my patients with pain, without whom this book would not have been possible.

Contents

About the Author

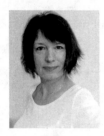

Jutta Richter

Dr. phil. Jutta Richter is a psychologist and physiotherapist; certificate Medical-Psychotherapeutic Hypnosis (Self-Organizing Hypnosis™ n. Renartz); certificate NLP; certificate Biofeedback-Therapy; certificate Brainspotting-Traumatherapy.

She has been working in her own practice in Bochum since 2004. Since 1995, she has been involved in various lecturing activities in the field of psychology and physiotherapy. She holds advanced trainings, courses and lectures on the topic of pain, stress processing and communication. One of her main research interests is the treatment of patients with chronic pain, diseases with psychological comorbidities and the effect of biographical and transgenerational experiences on pain and stress perception.

Preliminary Remarks

Multimodal pain management ...

If pain threatens to become chronic or already has, pain therapy will be necessary. It should ideally not only be one-dimensional, but multimodal, i.e. simultaneously on a bio-psycho-social level; i.e. it should include components from different disciplines that integrate biopsychosocial aspects:
- medical and pharmacological therapy,
- the psychological self-hypnosis
- pain therapy and stress reduction,
- physiotherapy, exercise and sports activities, and
- lifestyle and behavioral changes.

... is amazingly successful

Several years of studies in clinics and outpatient pain clinics show: A good cooperation of all disciplines with good cooperation of those who suffer from pain often achieves successful results with regard to the intensity as well as the duration of pain – especially if "psychosomatic" factors are included.

Nevertheless, it must be regretted again and again that multimodal treatment, especially accompanying psychological support, hardly takes place; suitable offers are still too few to be found. This applies in particular to the outpatient sector.

The book is essentially divided into three main parts:

Information

In **Part I**, information is given on the following topics: pain development and pain processing; what are the possible causes of persistent pain, and what are the goals of psychologically oriented pain management?

Methods and techniques

Part II is dedicated to the methods and techniques of psychological pain management. For this purpose, there are over 30 exercises on cognitive, emotional and body-awareness based modulations. Various relaxation procedures, self-instruction and attention guidance, mindfulness exercises and breathing techniques, imagination procedures and biofeedback are presented.

Changes at the behavioural level

Part III deals with changes on the behavioural level and how these can be psychologically motivated. Lifestyle and pain behaviour, such as dealing with stress, with insufficient physical exercise and one's own pain-reinforcing reactions are analysed. And constructive possibilities of relearning are shown.

Different therapeutic approaches

The techniques and exercises in this book are based on various therapeutic approaches and elements of the following procedures:
- Cognitive behavioral therapy,
- Relaxation methods and breathing techniques,
- Concepts of Mindfulness,
- Self-hypnosis and deep relaxation,

- NLP (Neurolinguistic Programming),
- Focusing (body- and experience-oriented therapy),
- modern, systemic and self-organizing hypnosis.

Before we start: In order to become clear about the space the topic of pain occupies in your own experience, you can carry out the following test.

Test: How Much Is Your Everyday Life Determined by Pain?

Contents

© The Author(s), under exclusive license to Springer-Verlag GmbH, DE, part of Springer Nature 2023
J. Richter, *Unlearn pain*, https://doi.org/10.1007/978-3-662-65702-7_2

■ ■ **Abstract**

This test will give you an idea of how much pain you feel, especially if it has been going on for a long time or if it can no longer be attributed to a definite cause.

This test will give you an idea of how much pain you feel, especially if it has been going on for a long time or if it can no longer be attributed to a definite cause.

Answer the questions below according to the following point system:

❯ **Rating**

Right: 2 points

True in part: 1 point

Not true: 0 points

Test questions about the pain load

1. I keep thinking about my pain all day long.
2. I do worry that there is some serious condition behind my pain.
3. The pain is affecting my life a lot. If the pain continues at this intensity, my life will no longer be worth living.
4. Because of the pain, I react much more irritably to my surroundings.
5. I often feel the need to be left alone. Because of the pain I retreat more and more into myself/out of social life.
6. I have to be careful and watch my movements carefully. Many movements and activities are affected by pain.
7. I'm so annoyed. Sometimes I fear that the pain is driving me out of my mind.
8. The pain deprives me of sleep.
9. I hardly know how to control my pain. I am a victim of my pain.
10. I often think about whether my pain will ever go away.
11. My performance and focus are quite impaired due to the pain.
12. If I had only found the right therapy/therapist, my pain probably would have been gone by now.

❯ When you have scored all the questions, add up your points.

Evaluation

0–7 Points

Evaluation of the test result

Pain is hardly a problem for you. You are not overly influenced by it. Either you have accepted pain as part of your personal life/age, or you have found suitable ways of reducing pain.

8–12 Points

You can tolerate your pain for the most part and are not constantly suffering from it. You probably know when your pain is getting worse and that you can reduce it by minimizing certain stressors in your life.

Learning relaxation techniques and pain management can help you prevent your pain from increasing in particularly stressful situations.

13–18 Points

Your attention, feelings and attitudes are strongly determined by the pain. Your hobbies, movements and (social) activities probably suffer. But these very activities could distract from the pain, they could reduce negative thoughts and stress.

Get out of this negative loop of pain – stress – fear of expectations! Learn again to take your life into your own hands, to consciously and purposefully influence your pain and to recognize your stress factors. Exercises in psychological pain management can help you to do this!

19–24 Points

For you, pain is a significant problem. All your thoughts and actions are governed by pain, and you have little hope that anything could change. Your life is so severely affected that you should seek external help: Discuss your problems with other people, and consult your doctor or psychotherapist. This should also clarify whether another illness, such as depression or anxiety disorder, needs to be treated as well.

Part I: What You Should Know About Pain

Contents

More than 14 million people are affected

Who does *not* wish to be healthy and pain-free. This desire can currently not be fulfilled for many people. According to various estimations, 14–20 million people in Germany live with chronic pain, i.e. pain that lasts longer than 6 months or recurs.

The suffering is often unimaginably great for the individual affected: constant pain wears you down, limits you, makes you despondent. Especially when the cause can no longer explain the high degree of pain and impairment.

Everyone knows pain, almost everyone rates it as unpleasant and wants to get rid of it quickly. In many cases, this also works out. Usually, when an acute injury heals, the pain decreases with it. Sometimes, however, the pain no longer corresponds to the corresponding tissue damage, i.e. it remains even after the healing process. Then one speaks after about 6 months of chronic pain.

Typical body areas

There are typical areas of the body that are prone to chronic pain. Back pain alone—especially the so-called "nonspecific back pain" without demonstrable or adequate organ damage—is already considered a widespread disease: every third German has it permanently, every second occasionally. Headaches and migraines, muscle and joint pain, nerve irritations, etc. are other pains that can become permanent.

Sometimes no organic cause

Sometimes, an organic or physiological connection can be found medically—sometimes not. In the latter case, it usually becomes difficult for the person concerned.

The Characteristic Path of the Pain Patient

Reduction of the quality of life

People with chronic pain often have a long odyssey through the offices of doctors and other therapists behind them. They experience several, sometimes futile or not permanently effective therapies. This always creates hope, which alternates with doubt and disappointment; at some point resignation sets in. Pain takes on a central place in one's life; all thinking and feeling revolves around pain and its effects. Social consequences (e.g. lack of understanding in the family or social environment), physical consequences (e.g. restricted mobility) and psychological consequences (e.g. feelings of isolation) intensify the suffering. The quality of life is perceived as increasingly poor.

If the pain cannot be clearly assigned organically or the region of pain changes constantly, those affected will at some point doubt their own perception.

Pain is always real …

Even today, chronic pain sufferers run the risk of being classified as malingerers by their environment, in case the doctor cannot prove any physical causes—and many sufferers eventually classify themselves as such. However, pain is experienced and felt in real terms—it is always "real".

The most difficult thing about pain is that you seem to have little personal control over it. The intensity and timing of its occurrence cannot be controlled, resulting in a feeling of helplessness. By avoiding movements, activities or situations that trigger pain, one tries to avoid the pain and, thus, to retain a certain influence. However, it is precisely this that often leads to an expectation of pain associated with fear, which one in turn tries to escape by further avoidance.

... and seems to be hardly controllable at all

Some sufferers feel bitter disappointment that they have now forfeited the physical integrity they had previously experienced due to the constant pain. The previously well-functioning body becomes an unreliable comrade due to episodes of pain, which then has to be fought or controlled rather.

Another aspect is that pain patients, despite multiple medical examinations, often still harbor a deep uncertainty about whether there is not a serious other, organic disease behind the complaints. This is associated with the constant question of whether everything has been discovered and everything possible has been done to heal the patient. This can also fuel fears.

Is there really nothing dangerous causing the pain?

What all sufferers have in common is waiting for some kind of miraculous cure. They hope that the pain will disappear as soon as they have found the right technique, the right therapy, the right cure.

Some people discover the right method for themselves— but much more often there is an endless chase from therapy to therapy—with the result of increasing disappointment. More effective and solution-oriented can be a real confrontation with the pain, combined with the change of unfavorable lifestyles.

People with long-lasting pain often compare their current physical state with times when they were still pain-free. The difference is usually immense. Such a comparison inevitably leads to feelings of disappointment and frustration. The positively remembered past is sometimes 20 or 30 years ago. It is forgotten that in the meantime quite normal ageing processes have also left their traces/marks in the body. And not rarely a memory also turns more positive over time compared to when the events were originally experienced ...

All too positive memories

Most patients with chronic pain expect a therapy to reduce pain a hundred percent . Disappointment is usually pre-programmed here. More realistic is a reduction of pain by 30–50%—if pain can be reduced even further, this is gratifying, but cannot be forced.

Expectations too high

A realistic goal can also be to maintain the current condition, i.e. to prevent worsening of conditions!

First and foremost, embrace the pain!

Acceptance of (remaining) pain is probably the most difficult challenge for people with pain. But this is exactly the very first goal. One could say it is a necessary prerequisite for successful countermeasures.

> ❯ The lower the unrealistic expectation of freedom from pain, the greater the likelihood of successful pain management.

Prerequisites for Pain Management

"Pain is an unpleasant sensory and emotional experience associated with (…) or without tissue damage." This is the WHO definition of pain. What is meant is that pain always has a physical and a mental component.

Biopsychosocial model of pain development

All modern pain theories today confirm the biopsychosocial model of pain development. This means that pain processing is always defined as a complex process that takes place both, on a *biological* level (in the body/central nervous system) and on a *psychological* (in thinking, feeling and behaviour) and *social* level (in interaction with others).

Therefore, it makes sense to deal with pain on a biological, but also on an emotional and social level. Those who see their pain purely in physical terms are falling short here.

Act actively and on your own responsibility!

The most effective changes happen when those affected by pain begin actively and on their own responsibility to recognize and help solve their problems. The realization that the most important lever for less pain is in one's own hands is new to many people.

At the same time, it is crucial to face pain as calmly as possible, not to classify it as a catastrophe, because it is not dangerous (to life). It is also important to understand that pain is to a certain extent part of life.

The brain can relearn

Learning processes are largely involved in a person's experience and perception of pain. In this sense, active pain management is a relearning process. Thanks to its flexibility, the brain can unlearn pain and learn how to deal with it. Similar to a perfume that you no longer smell after a while, chronic pain can also be filtered out of your attention.

This requires repeated practice of pain-relieving measures. The brain, nervous system and body, like a muscle, need to be well-trained to firmly establish behavioural change and pain relief. Such learning processes are best enhanced by making them fun and by ensuring that the desired goal is accompanied by high motivation. The stronger the desire for positive change and the more it is possible to actually bring about the change (processes), the more likely they are to be crowned with success.

Success is the best way to maintain or even increase motivation. Success comes only through "doing", preferably through repeated doing. Then the body can get used to new states and behaviors.

Success through motivation

Waiting for success, however, requires a certain amount of stamina. Obstacles or minor setbacks are inevitable and should be taken into account with understanding. It is just as important to take the time to then consciously perceive the successes, to perceive the changes, to acknowledge them and to enjoy them.

Be patient with yourself, change takes time! But don't succumb to the thinking error: You first have to wait for improvement, in this case for painlessness, so that you can then do something—it works exactly the other way round. This cannot be stressed enough!

Don't wait for things to get better before you do anything!

Even if you cannot believe in the effectiveness of individual techniques at first, keep an open mind and give them a try anyway—surprisingly, success often comes more clearly than expected.

One of the most important prerequisites for pain relief is, as already mentioned, the acceptance of one's own pain. This may sound contradictory. But only when the problem is perceived and acknowledged as such, one no longer needs to fight against it. That takes the pressure from/off the individual.

Instead of trying to avoid and push away the pain at all costs, space is then created for a neutral, rather benevolent observation:

Observe the pain as unexcited as possible!

— Under what conditions do I actually have pain?
— What makes them stronger? What causes them to weaken?
— What situations and countermeasures can I use?
— What initiative can I take myself—what is my responsibility, what are my options?
— Which behaviour or inner attitude can/must I change?

Sometimes it is also necessary to be honestly aware of the positive aspects of one's pain and to ask oneself what possible benefits the pain brings:

Benefits or conflicts of interest due to pain?

— What work can I avoid?
— What tedious tasks or decisions will I be spared?
— How much affection do I receive over pain?
— What other conflicts or problems in my life do I urgently need to clarify or resolve first?
— For example, what is the protective function of pain; what is different when I am pain-free?
— What other, even more unpleasant emotion or experience does pain prevent or displace?

It is striking—but the benefits of pain could then even outweigh and be the reason why the organism does not let go of the pain. Then you only get further if you are willing to learn to solve your underlying problems and communicate your needs differently, more maturely.

❯ If, despite intensive efforts, there is little improvement or if you find that your pain or problems cannot be solved by you in self-help, please seek help—e.g. from a doctor or psychologist. Do not see it as a defeat or your own fault if you have to resort to expert help.

Goals of Psychological Pain Management

What does pain management have to do with psychology?

When patients with chronic pain are offered psychological support, they usually initially think of it as a form of psychotherapy and tend to react sceptically because they experience their pain as being caused physically rather than mentally. Moreover, they do not want to be seen as psychologically impaired.

Psychological (co-)morbidities must be treated as well.

Psychotherapy for chronic pain sufferers can be very useful if the causes of the pain are predominantly psychological or if there are significant concomitant psychological disorders (e.g. depression, anxiety disorder, trauma, etc.).

Pain as a permanent stressor

Today, however, psychological pain management focuses primarily on the psychological consequences of long-lasting pain. Pain can be psychologically very stressful, it has effects on thinking, feeling, acting and acts like a permanent stressor on the organism.

The question is then: How can this permanent stress be reduced in such a way that a self-determined, relaxed life becomes possible again?

Control over the pain experience through psychological techniques

Psychological pain management techniques demonstrate effective and scientifically based ways to regain control over pain, increase pain tolerance, positively influence the experience of pain, and actively reduce pain. In doing so, psychological pain therapy works as a curative treatment where psychosocial factors are seen as causing or maintaining pain. For example, where other (e.g. biographical) stress factors exist and can be reduced or where unfavourable attitudes unintentionally increase pain, this is the case.

Life satisfaction increases

When psychological methods and techniques are successfully applied, the following medium- and long-term results are obtained:

▬ The perceived pain intensity is reduced.

- The frequency of pain attacks is reduced.
- Pain tolerance increases, the ability to tolerate pain is increased.
- Information on the development of pain and on biopsychosocial interactions leads to more understanding and greater acceptance of one's own pain.
- Unfavorable thinking patterns and emotional processing, as well as habits and behaviors that increase pain, are identified and modified.
- Cognitive, emotional, and behavioral strategies for pain management are learned and can be applied appropriately.
- Fears and feelings of helplessness regarding the pain are reduced, the possibilities of control increase.
- Mental resilience and psychosocial skills are strengthened in terms of stress management, problem-solving skills and communication.
- The body's own pain inhibition and self-healing powers are stimulated.
- Changes in exercise and health behaviors are implemented.
- The body feeling improves, the physical load capacity increases, the patient's confidence in himself and his body increases again.
- The quality of life, i.e. life satisfaction increases.

The primary goal of psychologically oriented pain management is not the elimination of the *physical pain* itself—this will occur as a consequence in the best case—but the relief of the *pain suffering*. What is the difference?

Pain relief

Pain always takes place on both, the physical-sensory and the mental-emotional level. One could say that there is no physical pain without accompanying feelings. Having a stabbing body sensation, for example, is usually not the problem in the first place—one can get used to it if it is not classified as dangerous. It is only when fear is added, for example of not being able to get rid of the body sensation in question and of being affected by it forever, that pain becomes unbearable. These cognitive-emotional reactions, such as accompanying thoughts, worries or feelings of threat, are what make up the experience of pain, the suffering. They can be influenced i.e. in the best case they can be unlearned.

Fear can be unlearned

Psychological pain management aims to make people aware of and change unfavourable pain triggers, pain processing mechanisms and lifestyle habits. Techniques for pain relief, stress reduction and relaxation are to be learned, the ability to solve problems is to be strengthened, own resources are to be tested, body and pleasure perception are to be trained. In addition, social activities and support are developed and movement behaviour is built up.

How does psychological pain management help?

Understanding Pain

Learning by insight

To approach the phenomenon of pain, it is advisable to understand it. How and through what does pain arise, how is it processed? As soon as something can be understood, it usually does not seem seem very threatening any longer. If pain is experienced as "meaningful" or at least as explainable, it is usually already reduced. And if you understand which factors intensify and maintain pain, you can develop appropriate solutions.

Pain is one of the most intense human sensations and can be terrible and beautiful at the same time. What does that mean? Injuries and chronic pain will certainly be counted among the most unpleasant sensations, while a birth or an athletic goal achieved in pain can be among the happiest moments in a person's life.

Different perception of pain

Strong motivation, a high goal, a sense of lack of threat, or an overlay of other sensations seem to completely block out pain perception.

In some cultures, initial rites that cause great injury are performed without the injured person perceiving pain.

Even in acutely life-threatening situations, pain is sometimes not felt. It would be "nonsensical" if thinking and feeling were dominated by pain while one has just fallen into a mountain crevice and is holding on to the rock with all of one's strength.

There are reports about severely injured soldiers in the military hospital who hardly complained about pain, but were glad to have gotten away with their lives. Pain is then simply not felt, it becomes secondary or even associated with something positive.

Pain is therefore evaluated very differently, depending on the experienced situation and expectation. The pain tolerance is just as individually different. No two people experience pain in the same way.

Individual learning story about pain

Everyone has a biography, a learning history about pain. Even a child makes painful experiences and perceives early on how its environment reacts to them. It learns how to deal with pain and also what pleasant aspects illness and pain can bring: The child receives comfort and attention, whereas those very demands are commonly not being met by the parents..

> Unfortunately, positively experienced effects have an unconsciously reinforcing effect on pain!

The biography of a pain patient very often shows particularly stressful life events—either currently or in the past. The extent to which these have a pain-intensifying effect must urgently be clarified or resolved beforehand. It is up to you to decide whether this is done with the help of your doctor or therapist. A solution makes sense in any case, because it clears the way for effective pain management.

The Pain System

Pain is basically not an adversary of humans, but a useful, life-sustaining damage early warning system. Without pain we would probably die. For example, it warns of the risk of injury, draws attention to tissue damage and to overuse or misuse of the organism. Pain then indicates a necessary change in behaviour. Most pain sufferers forget this aspect.

Pain as a useful damage early warning system

The pain processing system can be compared to a reporting system. Stimuli or pain triggers—e.g. damage of a mechanical, thermal or chemical nature—act on the organism. As a result, certain nerve fibres in the tissue are irritated. These pain sensors are called nociceptors and are located in the skin, organs, nerve roots and muscles. They react to the stimulus and transmit (or inhibit) impulses in the form of chemical messengers and electrical signals via designated nerve pathways to the central nervous system (CNS), which consists of the spinal cord and brain. The signals are received and processed in their individual control centres. Only when a certain amount of stimulus threshold is exceeded, or when inhibiting factors are switched off or overcome, is an excitation triggered in the pain centres and passed on to the brain. A very fast reaction then takes place in response to the message transmitted (e.g.: "Keep away from the hot stove!"). At the same time, the message of an incipient body damage ("Danger to the body!") is passed on to the brain. The transmitted impulses are then identified as pain, if necessary.

Notification only in the event of imminent danger

However, the pain only enters the consciousness of the person if it is classified as "dangerous enough" by the brain. Otherwise the message fizzles out, i.e. it is not consciously perceived. After all, 98% (!) of all transmitted impulses that could actually report pain are "inhibited" in this way by the body's own pain inhibition system, i.e. they do not enter the consciousness as pain perception. Simply because the system has not assessed them as dangerous or significant. However, the assessment of the threat to the organism is by no means objective, it is rather strongly dependent on psychological factors: the current mood of the person, the degree of attention or distraction or physical activity and, above all, it is dependent on the experiences one has had with pain so far.

Most pain stimuli are normally "inhibited away"

The central nervous system can therefore dampen the transmission of pain information through certain nerve messengers (neurotransmitters) and thus inhibit the perception of pain. One then "feels" no pain. However, this also means that pain is experienced when pain inhibition fails. In addition, the pain perception system can become overexcited or even permanently hypersensitive. In this case, even small stimuli that are per se harmless, i.e. that one would otherwise hardly notice, can be highly painful.

Physical and emotional pain are difficult to separate

Pain puts the entire nervous system on alert, a *physical* pain can hardly be considered separately from an *emotional* pain: because in fact the same (!) brain centers go into action and both types of pain processing in the brain are similar. Additionally, they reinforce each other. It can therefore be assumed that the arousal of the latter (e.g. through stress, negative experiences or fear of pain) also increases the arousal of the physical pain pathways. Emotional arousal thus increases the perception of pain. It is irrelevant whether the emotions are old, unresolved or currently explainable: The more stressed you feel, the more pain you actually feel. And the more pain, the greater the stress factor—a vicious circle …

Pain that Has Become Chronic and Its Causes

Chronic pain is more than the continuation of acute pain

Acute pain is when the organism reacts to (imminent) tissue damage with the appropriate pain; when the damage heals, the pain disappears.

Chronic pain, on the other hand, is pain that persists for more than 6 months despite organic healing and leads to suffering.

Often no clear cause (anymore) for the pain

The origins of chronic pain can be manifold, often no clear cause can be found (anymore), or the subjective symptomatology of the perceived pain and the organic findings hardly show any correspondence.

The realization of pain research in recent years is that pain can take on a life of its own. If there is no connection at all between pain and organic damage and the pain remains, one also speaks of an independent pain disease.

Thus, tissue damage with acute pain can become chronic pain if the once physical cause (e.g. wound, herniated disc) has been removed, the tissue has healed, but the pain remains continuous or recurs.

Nerve cells change

Then the nerve receptors in the body continue to report pain impulses to the central nervous system (spinal cord and brain). There, in response, more and more pain messengers are then released to the site of the pain. When the same stimulus is sent over and over again, the nerve cells also respond more and more over time. They become over-sensitized and also fire their signals uncontrollably to the brain. This process is comparable to an allergy with an increasingly strong sensitization to certain substances.

The constant irritation also changes the nerve cell itself, its biochemical metabolism and its structure. It then becomes more and more permeable for the pain messengers and reacts stonger and stronger. This once again intensifies the pain spiral.

The pain signals are led to certain centres of the brain. In response, these centres report increasing discomfort, a decline in mood and a drop in performance. Hormonal pain inhibitors and the body's own opiates, which could actually inhibit pain and improve one's mood, decrease as a result, with the consequence that pain is perceived more unchecked. One therefore reacts even more sensitively to new pain stimuli.

The changes in the nerve cells of the spinal cord can be so severe that there is even misinformation as a result of "short circuits" between two neurons that actually transmit different information (e.g. movement and pain impulses of a sensitive nerve). Thus, a simple movement can be converted into a pain signal. The body then falsely reports, "The movement hurts."

False News

Repeated, independent pain signals eventually leave memory traces in the brain, so-called engrams. These are quite firm connections of nerve fibres that achieve a stable memory of pain, in the same way that a muscle is trained through frequent exercise or a bad habit is almost impossible to break by means of frequent repetition. A pain memory has formed, the nervous system has learned pain, so to speak. The more similar the trigger situations are—they don't even have to be the same –, the faster pain is remembered.

Pain Memory

This also explains the phenomenon of so-called phantom pain: Limbs that have been amputated can continue to hurt because they are still represented in memory.

What further aggravates the process is that pain can actually displace areas in the brain that are actually responsible for other body regions or functions, e.g. for movement or touch. Instead of touch, pain is then experienced. Permanent pain also changes the perception of the body.

Changed body perception

Even if pain is felt on the body, it is "produced" in the brain or the central nervous system. So pain does not necessarily correspond to damage in the tissue, but to traces in memory. This is important for pain patients. This can put into perspective the concern that, for example, painful movements must be an indication of new injuries.

Pain originates in the brain

It is a current school of thought that we have a kind of gateway (as a metaphor) in the central nervous system. This can open to allow certain pain messages to pass if the brain interprets them as significant. Or it can remain closed, in which case the pain signals are blocked. For example, if we are very tense or anxious or suppressing feelings, the gate is more likely to open. If we are relaxed, distracted or in an optimistic mood, it is more likely to close and pain is less likely to be perceived. Experiences, moods and emotions have a decisive influence on the perception of pain.

No pain without muscle tension and vegetative reactions

Because we perceive pain as unpleasant, we develop fear and rejection of it; with accompanying negative emotions. Our mood drops and the feelings often have to be suppressed. The subsequent inner defense generates inner tension. Parallel to this, more or less strong muscle tension develops on a physical level. Then the feared pain sets in. These chain reactions play a significant role in the development of pain and the maintenance of chronic pain.

Pain researchers now agree that chronic pain is a highly complex process that is always based on a biological-psychosocial interaction whose components reinforce or inhibit each other.

Physical Causes of Chronic Pain

What physical factors tend to increase pain, and what can we do about it on a physical level?

A major cause of lasting pain is:

Consequences of physical inactivity

Lack of Exercise   The human body is designed for movement. But our everyday life often looks different: We sit too much and move too little. The modern lifestyle is a major cause of permanent muscle or joint pain in the postural and musculoskeletal system.

Too little exercise affects the entire body. Consequences are e.g. loss of strength and coordination of the musculature, thereby an incorrect use of joints, a reduced blood circulation of the entire organism up to metabolic changes, muscle tensions and tension dysbalances of the muscle-ligament apparatus.

Conversely, this also means that almost every pain experience can be positively influenced by movement!

Pain patients usually show a lack of movement behaviour, either originally—e.g. due to predominantly sedentary occupation—and/or as a consequence of the pain in the sense of movement avoidance. However, even less movement unfortunately leads to further negative consequences for muscles and joints and to a reduction in physical condition. One feels less well and morestressed at an early stage; the sensitivity to pain increases—whereby activity and movement are avoided even more.

❯ As a rule of thumb: half an hour of physical exercise daily (!) is a must.

Other physical causes of chronic pain include:

Incorrect Posture and One-Sided Stressful Activities Permanently one-sided activities or postures often lead to incorrect strain on muscles and joints. Consequences can be joint blockages, muscle tension and shortening up to wear and tear in the joints as well as damage to the intervertebral discs.

Most of today's occupations involve one-sided physical activities, which then result in hours of poor posture. People with pain often adopt relieving postures or tend to one-sided muscle tension, which on the long-term act like poor posture because they change the entire body statics (◘ Fig. 1).

Consequences of one-sided stress

❯ However, ergonomics can often be improved considerably by making just a few changes to the workplace!

For chronic pain can also be responsible, after all:

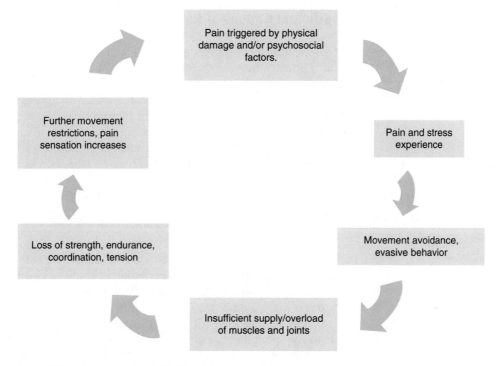

◘ **Fig. 1**   The pain cycle on the physical level

Other causes

Unfavourable Lifestyles and Their Consequences   In addition to obesity and/or an unbalanced diet as well as various addictions, a disturbed sleep rhythm or too little sleep is a particular burden on the organism. Almost all pain sufferers have a problem falling asleep or sleeping through the night—usually even before the onset of chronic pain. At some point, it is no longer possible to say what causes what. This is often followed by too little relaxation or an imbalance between effort and rest—another breeding ground for more pain.

On the other hand, persistent pain very often leads to sleep disorders. If you don't get enough sleep, you feel exhausted the next morning and even more sensitive to pain.

Pain patients often show a lack of body awareness of when they need a rest and relaxation. Particularly in phases with little pain, they want to be especially powerful, override limits and then put themselves under pressure.

However, it is precisely relaxation times that allow stress hormones, which stimulate the sensation of pain, to decrease again, thus having a pain-relieving and ultimately performance-enhancing effect.

❯ Relaxation phases and breaks are therefore not wasted time!

Medicinal Causes of Pain

Medical pain therapy also includes a well-adjusted medication. The attending physician will advise you on the type and frequency of medication to be taken.

Too many drugs

However, some people show an all too great willingness to take pain-relieving medication—even beyond what has been agreed on. In the right dosage, painkillers are sensible and necessary; yet, it is difficult to take them uncontrolled for too long or too much. Then medication itself can have a pain-increasing effect or create additional problems.

Other people are reluctant to take medication despite great pain, for example because they fear side effects. They only resort to it in extreme emergencies. However, if medication is only ever taken when the pain is very severe, this leads to a "reward effect" in the brain due to the subsequent freedom from pain in the body. On the other hand, it would be correct to take the pain medication adequately; the doctor in charge of the patient would be the best person to advise on this.

Too few drugs

Even if an increased willingness to perform is experienced due to the spontaneous pain relief achieved with medication, this can be perceived as pleasant. Nonetheless, an exaggerated increase in performance eventually leads to excessive demands!

Both set a negative learning effect in motion; on the long run, pain is thereby indirectly intensified.

Medications for pain relief can therefore contribute to the chronification of pain if taken incorrectly!

> ❯ A medicinal pain therapy absolutely belongs in the hands of an experienced physician!

Psychological Pain Amplifiers

Pain triggers not only physical but also psychological stress: Pain is usually accompanied by unpleasant feelings. Those who suffer constantly from pain inevitably change their mood, their thoughts and their behaviour. Persistent pain changes the perception, which becomes really fixated on the pain. Thoughts and feelings of threat, helplessness or even impotent rage are added. The affected person is often depressed, as he has lost his physical and mental integrity (❑ Fig. 2).

Such emotions, even if they are suppressed and hardly perceived, lead to increased physical stress reactions such as vegetative arousal and muscular tension. Avoidance of movement,

Fixation of attention on the pain

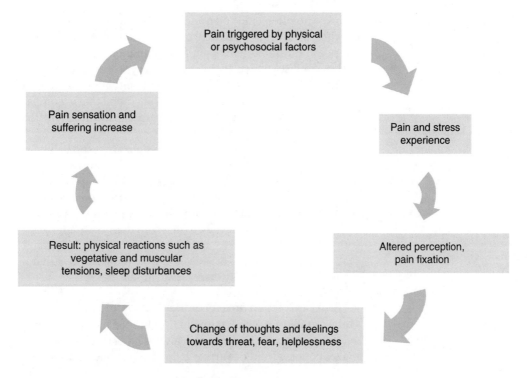

❑ Fig. 2 The pain cycle on a psychological level

relieving postures, sleep disturbances, anxiety and irritability are the result and in turn exacerbate the pain.

The chronification of pain is also promoted by additional psychological risk factors:

■ **Permanent Stress**

During exertion and stress, the body switches to "activity" and reacts with increased muscle tension. Permanently tensed up muscles cause a lasting muscle tension and, thus, ultimately pain.

Continuous pressure

Those who experience a high or permanent stress level, for example as a result of permanent everyday stress (such as a lack of job satisfaction, conflicts in the family and at work, a lack of social support, time pressure) or due to a difficult life event that still needs to be processed (such as death, separation, trauma, etc.), are under permanent pressure. Accordingly, recovery times are often short. Most of those affected report that they suffer more when they are under great daily stress and do something beneficial for themselves less often.

Negatively experienced permanent stress—especially if it is not sufficiently compensated—increases the perception of pain.

■ **Depressed Mood**

Pessimistic Mood

People who often tend to be anxious, depressed or pessimistic, or who suffer from boredom or feelings of loneliness, lower their pain threshold. One then feels pain more strongly under prolonged discomfort. It is therefore very worthwhile to look at one's inner mood. Not only on the one that occurs due to the pain, but especially on the underlying mood that accompanies us "always", quasi as life background music. Here the cause should be investigated if necessary.

Happiness hormones are missing

Changes in the nerve messenger system are responsible for the fact that pain is intensified. A depressed mood is accompanied by a reduced release of endorphins ("happiness hormones"), which have a mood-lifting effect and could dampen the perception of pain. In addition, a lack of endorphins in turn leads to a biochemically easier excitability of pain receptors. These are the nerve endings that receive and transmit pain information in the organism. So the implication is that a depressed mood actually increases pain sensitivity.

■ **Pain Expectation Anxiety or "Hang in there"**

Catastrophize

Unfavourable forms of individual pain management in turn aggravate the pain. Chronic pain always has a fear component, makes people afraid of further pain. This can increase to catastrophic thoughts: Perhaps there is a threatening cause for the pain; it cannot be controlled, I am helplessly at its mercy, I am worried about my future, etc.

Thus, pain can form an unhealthy alliance with feelings of fear, helplessness, and downright panic.

One then tries to avoid everything that could trigger further pain. This makes you tense and triggers further physical and psychological stress reactions.

Or one tries at all costs to suppress the fear of pain and attempts not to perceive pain. Activities are then increased despite great pain, whereby one tends to overexert oneself.

Pain suppression

Both attitudes are understandable, but in their extreme form they are unsuitable coping options. Avoidance of any stress as well as absolute perseverance "at any price" favors chronic pain on the long run.

On the other hand, those who find a way to remain mentally stable despite their pain, to exert a positive influence on their pain through self-care instead of anxious fixation, feel able to cope with their pain and thus their lives. This in turn increases pain tolerance and reduces the pressure of suffering.

Active pain management

In the case of long-lasting pain, psychological components of pain processing and adaptation do indeed gain in importance over time, so that a mixed picture of psychosomatic components is then present.

In addition, there are other psychological reinforcing mechanisms that induce or maintain pain, usually unintentionally.

■ Pain Creates Care

If the environment, e.g. the partner, is particularly compassionate or attentive towards you when you show pain (a gesture or facial expression indicating pain can be sufficient), this is unconsciously registered in the brain as a reward for the pain behaviour.

Attention as a reward

Unfortunately, this serves as reinforcement for the pain memory.

■ Pain Enables Withdrawal and Protection

Only when the pain becomes too much do we allow ourselves to rest or say no. Those who are ill and in pain need rest and cannot perform various tasks. Rest and being left alone is experienced as pleasant. The brain also registers this as a reward and can respond with pain when "everything becomes too much".

Spare time as a reward

Withdrawal can lead to the avoidance of movement tasks and social activities to such an extent that the vicious circle described above occurs: the more protection, the less activity, the more tense and untrained the body with its muscles, the quicker these very muscles will hurt or cause pain…

However, the opposite extreme of pushing oneself beyond the limit of performance on days with little pain also strengthens the development of pain in the long term.

■ Pain as an Accompanying Symptom

Body pain as an expression of mental pain

Body pain can of course also be an expression of past—mostly unconscious and repressed—emotional pain such as grief or anger. Further, it can be intensified if there is an underlying depression, anxiety or obsessive-compulsive disorder. It is estimated that between 30 and 60% of chronic pain patients suffer from a depression or anxiety disorder at the same time. This is where an experienced doctor or psychotherapist must make a diagnosis!

Pain caused by mental factors is just as real as other pain. Nevertheless, patients are always happy when the doctor finds an organic cause—even if this does not change the therapy at all.

How does pain management work?

So what is to be done? How can the risk factors mentioned be minimized, how can pain with its various causes be controlled and managed?

In short, how does pain management work, and how can it be practiced?

Part II: Exercises and Techniques for Pain Management

Contents

© The Author(s), under exclusive license to Springer-Verlag GmbH, DE, part of Springer Nature 2023
J. Richter, *Unlearn pain*, https://doi.org/10.1007/978-3-662-65702-7_4

Here are now presented individual techniques that you can perform as self-help exercises at home, possibly also on the road and at work. The exercises are described in a way that is easy to understand even for laypersons and are simple to implement; they require a little patience and alert attention; you need virtually no aids.

If you are still unsure, discuss the exercises with your doctor or therapist.

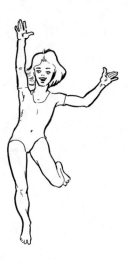

Instructions for Use

It is most effective if you first briefly skim the chapters to gain an overview. Then pick an exercise that particularly appeals to you and read through the text again thoroughly before using it. Try only 2–3 different methods per week, and be as focused on them as possible. It is of little use if all exercises are only briefly touched upon or are not followed through long enough.

Try only 2–3 different exercises per week

This way may seem cumbersome or tedious at first, but promises all the more success. Perhaps the number of exercises also seems too high to you. However, experience shows that over time you decide on 4–5 "favorite exercises", on which you then concentrate.

For all exercises:

— For most exercises, 10–15 min of daily practice time is sufficient.

Regular practice accelerates success

— Perform each exercise 3 times a day would be very effective.

— Regular practice speeds up success, irregular practice slows it down.

— If you can only practice very rarely, it is better to plan this time differently, because irregularly applied exercises hardly bring good results.

Everything you need:

— about 15 min of time, 1–3 times a day at convenient times,

— Paper and pen,

— a quiet, pleasant place,

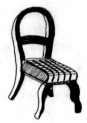

— Joy or motivation to practice,

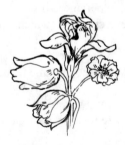

— Self-awareness and inner mindfulness.

At the end of a week, it is worthwhile to have a kind of retro-spective and then take stock: What worked, what didn't work so well? What do I still have to change?

The newly learned is still in need of protection

❯ Also consider that everything newly learned is like a "young plant" that wants to be protected in a certain way. Often the critical mind does not yet want to accept the new and possibly works against it. This becomes noticeable in inner sentences like "This won't stay so good, ... this can't work at all, ... maybe it's not worth the effort ...". Be aware of the critical voice in a friendly way – maybe it wants to protect you from disappointment – and then ask it patiently to step aside ...

The Pain Protocol

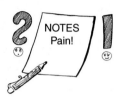

Before any work with pain, there is a pain analysis to determine when, how strong, by which triggers etc. pain occurs in the first place. pain occurs at all. The goal is a factual inventory, not an anxious fixation on the pain! It is best to take note of pain as calmly as possible and document it several times a day.

In the beginning, very short time intervals should be chosen, e.g. an hourly rhythm, in order to perceive the pain and the state of health. Later, after about 2–4 weeks, the intervals can be increased to 3 times daily documentation. After about 3 months, only the situations that trigger the pain are noted.

Some situations initially cause a certain inhibition against regular logging. However, you should make the effort to take notes even at work, in your free time, etc. The most important thing is first of all to make sure that you actually think about logging, e.g. by setting yourself an alarm clock or activating the mobile phone alarm. It is then also essential to link the exercises to fixed activities or times of day!

The purpose is a thorough pain analysis: when, how and by what exactly pain arises – or can be reduced. Pain conditions and changes are made conscious. The perception should become more balanced again. Instead of being one-sidedly fixated on pain, attention is shifted to well-being and beneficial exercises. Notice this and consciously take the time to enjoy it.

Perception becomes more balanced again

You may find that you have much more influence and control over your pain than you may have previously realized.

It is analysed and documented (more detailed explanation in later sections):

What is to be logged?

- the perceived intensity of pain,
- the duration of pain,
- the exact localization and spread,
- the accompanying symptoms (e.g., nausea, dizziness, muscle tension),
- possible triggers: situation, activity, circumstances,
- the correlating mood/state of mind at the moment,
- the severity of the impairment caused by the pain,
- the countermeasures used (e.g. exercises carried out, sporting activities, hobbies, relaxation, distraction; but also: good conversations, successful conflict resolution, source of stress minimised, etc.),
- the success achieved in terms of pain processing.

Successes become visible

It is astonishing that in many cases even a close observation of the pain leads to a reduction of the complaints.

Each record – as opposed to a loose memory – records the exercise-induced change in pain. A concrete basis for success is created, the written proof of improvement. This keeps you motivated, especially at times when it feels like you're treading water and making little progress – and progress will certainly come!

In addition, everyone can check themselves how regularly they do their exercises (e.g. relaxation, exercise).

Sometimes correlations show up surprisingly differently than expected when they are logged over a longer period of time – e.g. 4 weeks. The results found can then be analysed and possibilities for change sought.

Questions like these can be helpful:

Protocol evaluation

- Is there a recurring pattern per day/per week/per event or by certain activities?
- Are there interactions between tension and certain postures and pain?
- Is there a correlation between pain and tension on the one hand and thoughts (fears, stressful emotions) on the other?
- Instead of avoiding pain-increasing activities altogether, is it possible and reasonable to modify them?
- Can I also find activities that are more conducive to pain relief?
- Are changes (e.g., reducing the source of stress) addressed directly or cautiously?
- Or, if changes are not possible at the moment, where can at least an appropriate balance be found (e.g. through daily relaxation exercises)?

❯ It cannot be stressed strongly enough: Record your findings in writing!

Date	Time	Starch	Duration	Localization	Symptoms

Trigger	Mood	Impairment	Measures	Success

A copy template for a pain protocol can be found in the service section.

Implementation Here is a detailed explanation of each entry:

- **Pain Intensity**

Pain is very subjective and is always experienced differently. Therefore, the intensity of pain must be assessed individually and several times a day – and additionally at the beginning and after each exercise. The current value is determined on an imaginary or actual scale of 0–10 (where 0 means no pain at all and 10 means the strongest pain imaginable).

```
|__|__|__|__|__|__|__|__|__|__|
0            5            10   Pain level
```

- **Pain Duration**

How long has the pain lasted?

- **Localization**

Where exactly is the main pain, how far does it possibly spread?

Are there other pain zones, and where exactly are they located?

- **Associated Symptoms**

What other symptoms accompany the pain?

Are there changes in muscle tension, breathing, pulse, etc.? Is the pain accompanied by nausea, dizziness …?

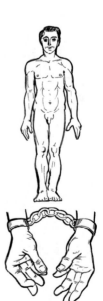

- **Possible Triggers**

What situation are you in right now? What activities, postures or circumstances can you identify that are associated with the pain?

- **Mood**

What thoughts, feelings and moods are accompanying you right now or have preceded the pain?

What thoughts and feelings does the pain trigger?☺ ☹

- **Impairment**

On a scale from 0 (not at all) to 10 (maximum), to what extent do you immediately feel impaired by the pain – e.g. in your movement, concentration, etc.?

■ **Countermeasures**

What self-help options (such as relaxation exercises, exercise, taking a break, mind control, etc.) can you think of and do you use?

■ **Success**

How successful were the countermeasures applied?

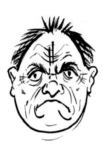 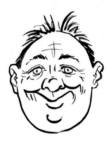

Now what is the pain level from 0 to 10 as a consequence?

> After each exercise used here or at the end of the day you should stop and ask yourself: What has done well, what has not yet worked so well? What still needs to be changed?

Change of Thinking, Evaluation and Attitude

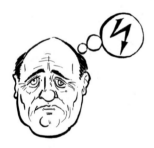

As described, stressful, unpleasant thoughts have a great influence on our experience of pain. Conversely, this means that serenity and pleasant thoughts have a pain-relieving effect. But what can you do when pain is distressing and accompanied by worry? Positive mood does not happen simply by wanting or making an effort.

You're going to have to deal with the pain.

The prerequisite for this is a closer look at the pain. Many people think that it will get worse if they pay attention to it. Despite all efforts, however, it seems that attempts at not wanting to think about pain fail miserably and produce ever more overwhelming thoughts and fears. It is not conscious attention to the pain, but repression, not wanting to acknowledge it, that creates feelings of helplessness and eventually a constant struggle. This costs a lot of energy and increasingly determines the thinking and feeling.

Take a closer look at your pain

It is more efficient to first consciously perceive and analyse one's pain in order to then look for suitable solutions. This usually has a very relieving effect, feelings of helplessness and loss of control are reduced, the fear of the problem of pain is reduced.

An analysis that is as precise as possible should identify unfavourable thoughts, evaluations and attitudes that increase pain and show what possibilities there are for change.

In the following exercises, psychological methods and possibilities of dealing with pain are presented. They involve thoughts, evaluations and feelings.

Exercise 1: Decoupling Body and Emotions

When we feel pain, on the one hand we receive information on the physical-sensual level: How does the pain feel physically, where exactly is it located, how strong is it to be measured, ...? On the other hand, these pain sensations are "coloured" by a mental evaluation – this happens involuntarily and immediately. The initially pure bodily sensation thus becomes emotional – the pain is e.g. unpleasant, unbearable, frightening etc.

It is useful to consciously separate these two levels for a while. Even if this seems somewhat artificial at first, it is often surprising how little actual physically felt pain there can be – the added feelings of fear, threat or frustration, however, are what make it so distressing.

Implementation   At the beginning and after the end of the exercise, the current pain level on the pain scale is assessed.

The exercise is divided into four phases:

▪ Phase 1: Rating
The current pain is felt and the exact pain intensity is determined according to the pain scale of 0–10. How strong is my pain right now?

Determine pain intensity

▪ Phase 2: Observing the Body
At first, only the physical-sensory sensations are noticed and considered as calmly as possible: "Aha, the pain is probing, feels hot, is just below the right kneecap, has an intensity of 6 at the moment ..."

Observation of physical sensations

▪ Phase 3: Observing Emotions
Then, as accurately and factually as possible, the feelings and evaluations that arise are noticed and described: "It scares me that the pain might not go away ... I'm angry that I now have to cancel my appointments ... I'm gradually losing hope for improvement ..." etc.

Observation of emotions

Pendulum between feeling
and body

■ **Phase 4: Commuting**

Stay once for about 1 min (this corresponds to about 8 calm breaths in the direction of the abdominal region) on the physically felt level (phase 2) – then switch to the emotional level (phase 3) and perceive your corresponding feelings for about 1 min.

Repeat this process about 2–3 times, swinging back and forth between these two levels and perceiving each as accurately as possible without evaluating them. Then feel for it.

At the end, as at the beginning, there is always the question about the current pain intensity (scale 0–10). What changes have you noticed?

❯ It is amazing how much a factual-distanced perception can reduce the physical pain (sensory level) as well as the suffering (emotional level). Feelings of powerlessness and helplessness will change!

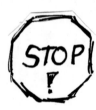

Exercise 2: Thought Stopping Technique

Thoughts are supposed to keep our minds clear and solution-oriented. Sometimes, however, they become downright worries due to accompanying emotions such as fear, anger, etc.. Then they are not very constructive and end up in repetitive thought loops. When thoughts no longer lead to a goal and possible solutions, they should be stopped. This can be done by sensory stimuli and other distractions. Especially loud or "surprising" signals are suitable for this.

■■ Examples
— Auditory signals (listening): shouting "Stop!" or "Halt!" loudly or clapping hands,

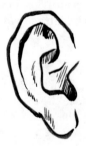

- visual signals (see): suddenly hold the palm of the hand in front of the eyes like a shield,

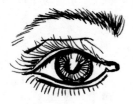

- sensitive signals (feel): grasp the wrist with a firm grip,

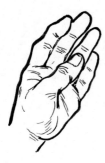

- olfactory cues (smell/taste): smelling lemons, sucking ice cubes.

Implementation Take a rating of your pain on the scale of 0–10 before and after each exercise process.

The exercise is performed in three steps.

■ Phase 1: Analysis of Thoughts

Whenever you notice that your pain is pulling you into unconstructive ruminations, become aware of these thoughts: What thought is keeping me going right now/lately?

Concentrate on this thought and let yourself go with it for a moment. Does the thought take shape? Then say loudly in a command tone: "STOP!", or you suddenly and as intensely as possible use one of the counter-stimuli mentioned above.

This should stop the mind spinning.

Repeat this step 3–5 times, making sure that on each pass you actually let the disturbing thought come up and only then interrupt it.

Consciously perceive brooding

■ **Phase 2: Change of Activity**

Change activity spontaneously

The next step is to change your current activity: If you are currently walking, stop now. If you are quiet right now, sing. If you are tensing your face right now, now smile …

■ **Phase 3: Activation of Positive Thoughts**

Activate pleasant thoughts

Immediately you should consciously put pleasant thoughts in the gap created by the interrupted brooding: Think of a loved one, recall a pleasant situation, focus on the beauty of the landscape around you …

Practical Tip

The various stop stimuli can also be combined to possibly increase the effect of distracting from brooding. They can also be performed inwardly, i.e. in the mental imagination. However, they must be strong enough to initiate a thought interruption.

■ **Variation**

You can also take a little detour:

Slight detour

Negative thoughts and feelings are again consciously allowed for a time. In doing so, you should adopt an attitude of acceptance: The thought is appreciated, i.e. neither negatively evaluated nor pushed away. You can let it play out like the scene of a movie. You watch everything as a spectator from some distance. Stay with it for 1–2 min.

Then the thoughts are actively sent away, this can be well achieved by inner imaginings.

Choose one of the following examples:

– Imagine disturbing thoughts floating away like balloons.

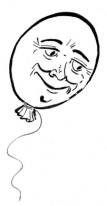

— Wrap the thought/problem in your imagination, bury it, burn it or destroy it.

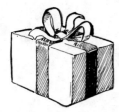

— Invent/remember a nice, safe place miles away from here and give your problem/disturbing thought there.

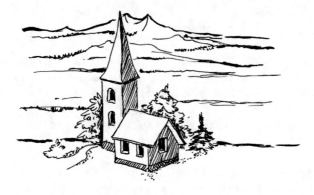

▶ During the first day or two, the frequency of disturbing thoughts may even increase by using a thought-stopping technique. But hang in there! This will regulate itself, and after three days at the latest, your brooding will be significantly reduced until you are finally hardly affected by it anymore.

Perseverance pays off

Exercise 3: Redirecting Attention

Pain can be moved into the perceptual background by distraction. This can be compared to perfume, which we no longer smell after a while, or a continuous sound, which we notice less and less as we get used to it – because it is filtered out of our attention. We then no longer perceive the pain.

By distraction ...

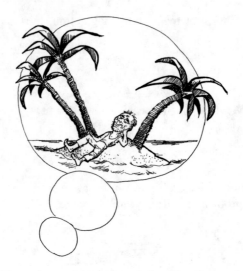

... the perception of pain can be reduced

Also, when we are in love or looking forward to something, we are distracted and feel less disturbing. Distraction that makes positive feelings reduces pain. Take advantage of it!

Implementation   At the beginning and after the end of the exercise, the current pain level on the pain scale is assessed.

When pain occurs, always consciously put yourself in a pleasant situation and direct your attention to it as much as possible:
    Choose one of the following examples:

New connections through pleasant experiences

— Focus on a real situation or consciously notice the beautiful surroundings. Surround yourself with pleasant people or do something good for yourself here and now.
— Consciously change everyday situations, give new impulses to everyday routines: choose different ways of working, change meal times and familiar routines so that they become interesting and enjoyable again.
— For once, abandon your usual planning – at first, until you have gained more courage, in areas that are not dangerous – and get involved in the situation in a completely new way, which now requires your full attention.
— Focus on a mental image, such as a fond memory, an imaginary landscape, or a constructive solution to a problem.
— Focus on an activity that fully engages you and is experienced as pleasant by you: Your (new) hobby, singing, dancing, physical exercise …

Through repeated coupling of pain and pleasant or new, interesting experiences, the brain learns new associations over time. When this succeeds, the dangerous, unpleasant component of pain fades into the background because it has been filtered away. The brain has then relearned.

Exercise 4: Pain as a Counterpart

One way to take away the horror and diffuse existence of pain is to "personify" it. Of course, this seems funny or absurd at first. It is also good if you can take the pain with humor.

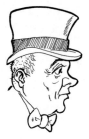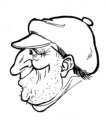

Implementation   At the beginning and after the end of the exercise, the current pain level on the pain scale is assessed.

- Take some time and leisure at the beginning. Now imagine your pain as a person with whom you can start a conversation … If necessary, keep a safe distance inside, so to speak, take a few steps back in your imagination.
- Like another person, take a good look at your pain, describe it, and give it a name.
- Describe to him your feelings, your emotions. Shout – actually or inwardly – your anger at him!
- Or approach him like a loving mother approaches her child. Reach out to him or praise him when he is less noticeable.
- Ask him to help you, or negotiate compromises to help him cope. Ask him what he might need from you, or what other need might be hiding behind it. And listen carefully!

Think of your pain as a person

Listen carefully

Allow one, or better still 2 min for each action, question or answer, so that they can trace it clearly!

This exercise will be very beneficial. It distances from the pain, makes constructive, attentive and promotes acceptance of pain.

Exercise 5: Change of Perspective

Every day we take in millions of old and new impressions with our organism, for the most part this happens unconsciously. These impulses are evaluated, sorted, processed and stored in memory. The way we see the world is made up of these impulses. In order not to overload the system, information is simplified and reduced. And because it has always been more

The way we look at our world is crucial

important for survival to notice (and adjust one's behavior to) when something is not going well, the organism is calibrated to dangers from the environment, to mistakes and stress factors, etc.: So it is more likely that deficits are perceived and stored as memories.

Now, unfortunately, one tends to think that only what one perceives is true. If mainly unpleasant things like pain are perceived, all thoughts and feelings fixate on them and the whole life seems painful.

Beautiful, joyful experiences sometimes fade into the background and are hardly noticed.

The suggestion to you now is to also experience the world differently, consciously in a positive way. The objective is to turn to pleasurable, even seemingly small things.

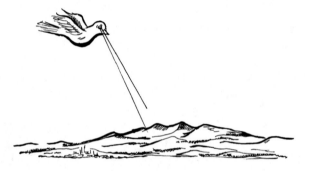

Get to know other perspectives

This is not self-deception or untruth, but rather an expansion – you will get to know situations from other perspectives. The more good experiences you have, the better you will feel. For this it will be necessary to experience the world in a more differentiated way than before, to consciously perceive the positive in a condition in addition to the negative.

Implementation Take a rating of your pain on the scale of 0–10 before and after each exercise process.

Choose a solution-oriented view

In any unpleasant, painful situation, one can ask:

— What seems to be the missing positive side of this situation?
— What good function does the unpleasant thing have for me: Do I also gain something from it? What does it protect me from, what can I do through it or what do I not need to do?
— How would I assess the situation from another perspective: What would the problem look like from a bird's eye view or from another person's perspective?
— How to make the best of the situation now?
— How will I judge the present situation, say, in ten years' time, or in the future when the problem has been solved?

- What would I have needed – looking back from the future – in the problematic situation, what was missing? And: How could I fill or solve this deficit **now**?
- How would I evaluate the situation if I were (otherwise) perfectly fine?

In a problem or pain situation, choose one of the examples mentioned. Find another perspective and get distance, this creates an inner open space. The pain can then attack you less.

Exercise 6: Affirmations: Formulaic Resolutions

Affirmations have the task of strengthening or realigning thinking, inner attitude and self-confidence.

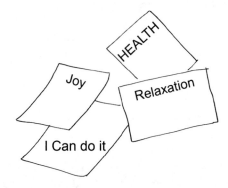

Affirmations are self-chosen, appropriate guiding sentences that one recites to oneself inwardly several times a day or during a relaxation exercise, experiencing them as intensely as possible. An ideal goal is named, which should be formulated positively and in the present. Thus, "I may feel a little better from day to day" instead of "I will have no more pain." In the case of great resistance – e.g. feelings of scepticism or shame – you can preface it with: "Even if I can't believe it yet – I'm getting a little better every day."

Affirmations can help to strengthen positive thinking and reduce negative thoughts and brooding over time. The first successes appear after 2–4 weeks.

Choose a suitable set

Implementation   To use it, first label some slips of paper, each with a positively worded sentence. You deposit these slips of paper in clearly visible places that you frequently visit, e.g. on your desk, on the mirror, on the front door, etc. After a few weeks you will no longer need the notes as a reminder. The guiding principles work mainly in the subconscious, i.e. even if you do not (yet) believe in their content with your mind. It is most effective to feel the affirmation completely for a moment, to let yourself be touched by it as if it were already reality.

Formulate a positive sentence

Here are some suggestions that you can adopt or adapt for yourself:

- "I know the pain will pass."
- "I get support from ..."
- "If I keep up ... (e.g. the relaxation exercises), the pain gradually reduces."
- "I stay calm and relax."
- "I can do it!"
- "Joy and confidence accompany me in ..."
- "I'm allowed to get better and better."

If necessary, put the following sentence in front of your affirmation, "Even though I can't believe it yet ..."

It's amazing: even if you are not yet convinced, your body and thoughts will follow the affirmations after some practice. – By the way, this also works the other way round: If you keep telling yourself: "I can't do this!", you are guaranteed to lose courage over time ...

Exercise 7: Cognitive Reappraisal: The ABC Model of Emotions

Humans have a constant impulse to evaluate themselves and their environment. We do this many thousands of times a day – often unconsciously. Through our mental evaluation of internal or external circumstances, we immediately judge them as pleasant or unpleasant, dangerous or harmless, positive or negative. These evaluations and thoughts that we direct towards something trigger feelings and a certain mood in us. As we know, mood has a significant influence on our perception and (pain) experience (◻ Fig. 1).

Notice how often you notice rather unpleasant thoughts and negatively colored evaluations about yourself.

On the other hand, how often do you feel comfortable and relaxed, how often do you experience internal or external circumstances in a more positive way? What is your balance?

Evaluations and thoughts trigger feelings

Then check how certain thoughts, e.g. of angry, discouraging, sad or even calming, encouraging situations, affect your body and muscle tension. You will notice: Just the thoughts and the associated feelings can trigger tension and pain.

Conversely, this means that when thoughts and evaluations are changed, feelings and moods also change!

People with chronic pain understandably tend to evaluate pain in an exclusively negative way. However, through a negative

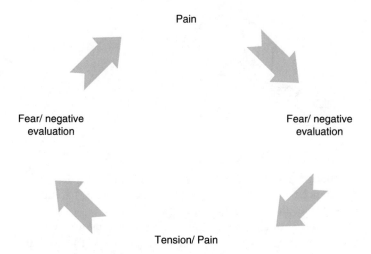

Pain

Fear/ negative
evaluation

Fear/ negative
evaluation

Tension/ Pain

◘ **Fig. 1** The cycle of pain and fear

mental evaluation (e.g.: "Pain is a threat!") our alarm system is ramped up. This is followed – sometimes imperceptibly – by further muscle tension, release of stress hormones, breath holding etc.. Usually this means an intensification of the pain.

You could almost say: The (unpleasant) meaning we give to pain has an effect on our feelings, or: Without negative evaluation we would hardly get into stress or pain suffering.

Unpleasant feelings can increase pain

How can this cycle be broken?

The goal is to change the negative thoughts towards more helpful, constructive attitudes.

Negative thoughts and evaluations that are immediately present must first be made aware of. They are there anyway, so ignoring them would be nonsensical. This perception works best if the thoughts are first accepted as objectively as possible and without an immediate tendency to reject (!) them. In a second step, they can be reflected upon and replaced or supplemented by more constructive evaluations.

Negative thoughts can be reworded!

This requires accepting introspection and some patience with yourself.

Implementation   At the beginning and after the end of the exercise, the current pain level on the pain scale is assessed.

The revaluation takes place in three phases:

■ **Phase A: What Is the Initial Situation?**

You are in a certain situation. Define as precisely as possible: What specifically are the circumstances? Events in themselves are neutral to begin with, that is the factual aspect that needs to be filtered out.

Initial situation

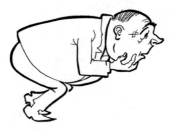

■ **Phase B: How Do I Evaluate this Situation?**

Mental evaluations

A situation does not remain neutral for us for long. Memories, experiences and associations immediately lead to certain thoughts, evaluations and meanings.

Typical thoughts and evaluation patterns include devaluing, dismissing, generalizing, self-pitying, exaggerating, blaming, etc.

These can be noticed – for example as an inner image or as an inner dialogue. The question is: How do I evaluate and judge this event, what goes through my mind?

■ **Phase C: What Emotional Reactions**
   Does this Trigger in Me?

Emotional response

The evaluation of the event leads quasi-automatically to a reaction, recognizable as a feeling, as a mood, and then subsequently as behavior. To perceive these, you might ask yourself:

What feelings arise in me, how does the evaluation affect my mood, how do I feel now? And what action/behaviour does this trigger in me?

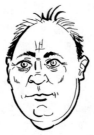 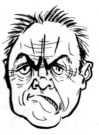

■■ **Example 1**

(A) *Initial situation:* I have a lot of work.

(B) *Mental evaluation:* I'll never make it! I will fail.

(C) *Emotional reaction/mood:* pressure, irritability, resignation.

■■ **Example 2**

(A) *Initial situation:* I have severe pain, scale intensity 7.

(B) *Mental evaluation:* This is becoming unbearable. I am powerless.

(C) *Emotional reaction/mood/behavior:* Helplessness, resignation and withdrawal.

■ **How Do You Solve This Automatism?**

After you have noticed and perceived the individual phases (without wanting to suppress them), you take a few steps back inwardly and create distance for yourself. Then consciously analyse the parts (A), (B) and (C) separately:

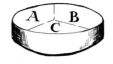

(A) What specifically is the circumstance/situation?

"The specific situation is that I have a lot of work/pain at this moment."

(B) How do I evaluate and judge it? What coloring does it have for me? Which thoughts follow automatically?

"I evaluate the situation negatively, as threatening; worries about the future overwhelm me."

(C) How do I react? What feelings are surfacing in me? How does this affect my mood?

"I feel overwhelmed, I react irritably/resigned."

Through the following step, a *cognitive re-evaluation* can now take place.

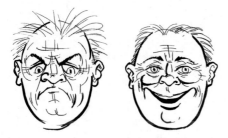

The key is to change the way you evaluate this situation. Questions like these can help:

— Could the rating be a little less negative?

— Now what would be even worse in this situation?

— Could the problem be seen less as a threat and more as a challenge? Or could there be a positive long-term goal?

- What would be solution-oriented? How could we make the best of the situation now?
- Was there a similar situation that could already be mastered – how did I succeed back then? How can it succeed now?
- Also, is there anything meaningful or humorous about this situation?
- Where have there been small successes, what has already been achieved – can I enjoy this?
- Who or what could be of help to me now? What possible solutions would another person suggest?
- How will it feel when the problem/pain will be overcome?

Example

In terms of a pain situation, that could mean:

"The current pain isn't pretty, but it's not hopeless either. I could try to help myself with heat and exercise, that has helped before." Or, "Pain is unpleasant, but never dangerous. Here's what I can do to influence it …"

Reverse a negative rating to a positive one

A sober situation analysis creates the necessary distance and often the possibility to turn a negative mental evaluation into a positive one. Realize once again that your *attitude* and *evaluation* determine your feelings and your behavior! A change of the evaluation would mean that then also changed (emotional) reactions would follow! Such a re-evaluation does not always succeed (immediately), but you should make in any case.

It is possible to change your thought patterns in the long term.

As a rule, patterns of evaluation and thought have become ingrained over many years. Fortunately, it does not take quite so long to change them, although one should always keep in mind that it is possible in principle to change one's neuronal circuits, i.e. to relearn. However, this is a process, and it takes about 18–24 weeks for this to become stable. Then your feelings and moods should respond to the changed thoughts, and that means: you will also feel better! This in turn will lower your pain level considerably – provided you practice and apply it regularly in everyday life, especially in pain or problem situations.

Do-as-you-go technique

Variation The effect of reappraisal can be enhanced by an anticipated positive association that is linked to the pain. That is, as soon as pain appears, we consciously emotionally associate it with pleasant experiences by acting as if *we were already in* a good mood, pleased or relaxed.

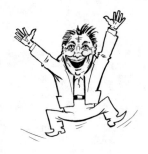

To do this, go into a pleasant situation in your imagination or remember earlier, positively experienced situations. Feel for this moment as if the pain/problem had already been solved. Experience this for a moment as intensely as possible, with all your senses … Then feel: How does it feel now? How has the pain changed?

This sounds absurd at first. But you will experience that the pain fades into the background.

The amazing thing is that the brain actually accepts this new association – if it is used intensively and frequently enough. After about 10–20 so-do-as-if reassessments, the brain has actually relearned!

Take influence on your thoughts and thus on your feelings! Even if the process of relearning seems strenuous – which it undoubtedly is: Negative evaluation, however, leads to unpleasant feelings and moods, is destructive – and intensifies the pain.

Take self-determined influence on your thoughts

Change of the Experiencing: Body Perception

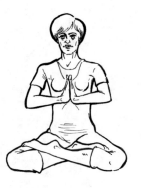

How does it feel inside me? How do I perceive my body, my feelings, my movements?

The ability to consciously feel one's body, one's senses and one's own actions is an important prerequisite for any self-reflection – and a prerequisite for holistically oriented pain management.

This ability to perceive the inner self, to feel one's own body and sensations, is sometimes lost in adulthood. And people with pain often avoid it. Fortunately, however, it can be remembered, trained and strengthened, in short: learned again!

Exercise 8: Training Mindfulness and Inner Perception

Conscious perception is a pausing, a concentrating on, an acceptance of the moment. It happens through the sensory channels and in the body: it means to see, hear, taste and smell consciously and mindfully, to feel oneself in one's body, one's movements, one's feelings, sensations and moods.

In mindfulness we "decelerate" a situation, thus counteracting stress and hecticness. In mindfulness we are open to the senses, as if we were experiencing the situation for the first time – not strained, but rather light and playful.

Conscious perception means pausing

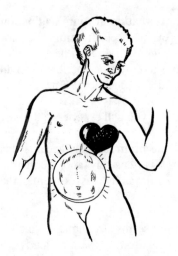

The right time is the "now"

We easily overlook the mindful experience in the here and now in everyday life. Many people do not even realize that they are exclusively "in other times". It is dwelling in the past or in the future – instead of in the present. In the future, we try to find a better feeling than the present one. Or we are doing well, and actually we could be happy and enjoying it. Instead, we think back to an event that went badly or a painful situation, so the joy dissipates. In the present we are usually in the right (pleasant and unpleasant) time – but we have to accept it.

It is one of the habits of our everyday behavior to be largely un-attentive. Many actions are done quasi automatically. This is partly justified, because not every activity can be thought through again and again. However, by doing so we also ignore the perception of our state of mind, ignore our body signals and stick to harmful behaviours. If we want to change behavioural habits, we must first recognise and gently perceive them.

Focus on *one* aspect

But how can mindfulness be learned or developed? Let yourself in, concentrate completely on *one* aspect of a situation or on one body-sense channel. Without tensing up, all feelings are allowed, thoughts can be perceived – and let them move on.

Implementation   At the beginning and after the end of the exercise, the current pain level on the pain scale is assessed.

Everything can be accompanied mindfully

Mindfulness can be incorporated very well into normal everyday life. Any activity can be accompanied by mindfulness: standing, walking, sitting, talking on the phone, professional activities, housework, etc.

Questions like these help:
— What am I doing right now, how am I doing it, and how do I perceive it?
— How does it feel in my body?

- How does it smell, how does it taste, what can I see, hear …?
- What thoughts/emotions accompany the situation?
- How do I evaluate it? Do I find it pleasant – or unpleasant?

You can also do everyday activities in a completely different way than usual: at a different time, with the other hand, by taking a different path or in a different order, etc. Then mindfulness succeeds quite easily. Then mindfulness succeeds quite easily.

Every posture, every body movement, every environmental stimulus can be grasped attentively and perceived sensitively. This directs the attention to alternative sensations instead of pain.

Mindfulness has a relaxing and stress-reducing effect, lightens the mood and reduces pain. This has been confirmed by neurophysiological research. Try it out – even with seemingly banal activities.

Mindfulness is easy to do

Exercise 9: Pleasure Training

The so-called pleasure training is a targeted attentiveness to positively experienced sensory impressions, to our strengths and resources. In everyday life, the focus tends to be on what is critical and still flawed. There is too little time and space for pleasant sensations. Often we no longer know what is good for us. Even when something desirable has been achieved, we hardly ever pause, but rush on to the next goal. Sometimes we really have to learn again what our own strengths and preferences feel like – and how to enjoy them.

Strengths and resources

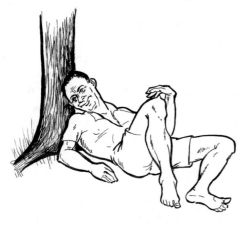

Enjoyment requires conscious sensual perception of beauty in our surroundings, of (even seemingly small) things or situations that create joy and balance. It needs conscious inner attention and time. Enjoyment is not something that can be done on the side!

Enjoyment needs sensual perception

What's good for me?

Implementation   Take a rating of your pain on the scale of 0–10 before and after each exercise process.

The following questions can support the perception process:

- What do I like – who or what is good for me: which situations, which things, which people?
- What do I succeed in doing well? What pleasant feelings accompany this success?
- How can I do something good for myself now?
- Sensory Experiences: What *does* my favorite … look like, what does my favorite … *smell like,* what does my favorite … *taste like,* what does my favorite … *sound* like, what does my favorite … *feel* like?
- What things in my life do I feel gratitude for, who/where can I be grateful to in this matter?
- What did it feel good to me before – how did it feel when there was no pain? When and in which situations was that? Can I remember this feeling with all my senses – and enjoy it?
- How would it feel if the pain had already subsided, the problem solved (at least a little)?
- Go on an inner quest:

How do joy, serenity, strength, gratitude, forgiveness … feel inside me?

Taking time to experience things, to acknowledge one's own resources has a relaxing and pain-relieving effect. And it creates a positive mood, a real buffer for the experience of pain.

Exercise 10: Mindful Focusing: Experiencing the Body's Knowledge

Inner Resistances block us

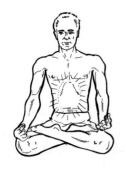

Sometimes it is not enough to reorganize one's inner evaluations and thoughts, because too strong aversion or feelings always again stand in the way. If you look for the positive or want to avoid the negative – if you actually want to eat less or smoke less, exercise more, etc. – then the knowledge of better health is indeed present. But inner resistances, which are stronger – or need infinite strength to be overcome – still prevent the implementation.

These resistances – which are perceived as negative feelings or pain – need to be traced. Through allowance and deep understanding they can often be dissolved.

This first requires the willingness to approach one's own pain – and also one's inner resistance – and to want to understand and feel it. This is already a great challenge, as one usually does everything to push pain away.

Implementation At the beginning and after the end of the exercise, the current pain level on the pain scale is assessed.

Solve resistance

- Take a few minutes and inner peace […].
- Get in touch with your pain/feeling: Focus on the inside of your body […], on your body feeling, the well-being or discomfort inside you […]. This is usually best felt in the abdomen, chest, throat or pharynx.

Get in touch with your pain

- Wait calmly for what comes up. At first, just welcome it with a calm inner attitude, even if the feeling is an unpleasant one […].
- If several pressing feelings/pain are perceived, choose the most pressing one first […].

Find a term for it

- When you have focused on a feeling/sensation, stay with it for a moment. How does it feel […]?
- When you look at it, can you find a *term for* it? For example, a suitable name, a title or a picture – it looks like …, it somehow feels like … […].
- Wait quietly until something suitable comes up […] – Is that the most precise term now […]?
- When you find the description that fits your experience, you get a feeling of distinct relief. It's as if you've just thought of a word that had been on the tip of your tongue for a long time.
- Now wander from the found concept back to your body sensation and stay with it for a while […].
- Then check: Does the term still fit exactly – or would I have to change it somehow […]?
- Direct your attention further inside the body (abdomen, chest, throat) and stay focused on the discomfort […]. Where exactly in the body is the sensation felt most strongly […]?

Where is the pain felt the most?

- Linger there for a moment, and feel them as consciously as you can […].

Consider this sensation with all your senses:

- What exactly does it look like, what *colour* could it be and what *shape* would it have? What *material* could it be made of, what temperature would it have […]?

What does the pain look like?

- What *sound*/tone or melody comes to mind […]?
- Does a *smell* or taste come to mind […]?
- How does it feel overall in my body, what *mood* does that create in me […]?
- What is the worst, the essential thing about it […]?

What is the essence?

- Do I know this pain/problem from other, perhaps earlier situations? What comes to my mind […]?
- What would it take now to make me feel a little better […]?

■ **Variations**

Choose one of the following examples:

Create free space
- When feelings or pain arise very violently, it is worthwhile to first create an inner distance. This gives you the space you need to avoid being overwhelmed by them. To do this, take a few steps back inwardly, or "push" the inner image a little further away so that you can look at it more calmly.

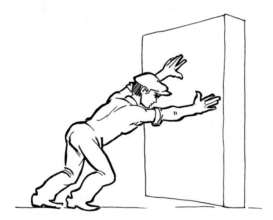

Role reversal
- Role reversal can also be very useful: imagine that the sensation/pain comes in the form of a person with whom you can communicate.
  - What would this person look like […]?
  - What would she say […]?
  - What would it feel like from their point of view […]?

Support
- Or you imagine a helping person who accompanies you in this situation: What support can he/she give me […], what advice […], how does the problem feel now […]?

■ **Practice Completion**

Solution questions
If you have perceived the situation in a differentiated way, then ask the problem/pain the following solution questions:
- What would you need to feel a little better […]?
- What would this feeling/problem need to be fully resolved? And what are the obstacles to this?
- If the problem/feeling stems from the past: What would it have taken at that time in the remembered situation […]?
- How would it feel if the situation was overcome, the problem/pain already solved? […]?

— What would I have to change in the future? What should I do, what should I no longer do [...]?

What would be good for the problem now?

Create different solutions and use one or two of them! Modulate your future behaviour (or feeling) in your imagination until the thing is coherent for you personally and feels good – take your time with it [...]!

Then slowly say goodbye [...]. Feel for a moment the feeling that comes when something is done or overcome [...]. Do you feel gratitude or joy?

Enjoy this state

Feel with all your senses – and enjoy this state for at least 2 min.

At the end it is useful to secure the successful process. Find something to remind you of the result achieved: write it on a card or in a (pain) diary, draw a suitable picture or find a symbol – and deposit it in a clearly visible place!

Securing the successful process

Reactivate your positive experience again and again – at least once a day.

> The sensing of sensations succeeds best when the entire attentiveness – without inner impatience, drivers, correction – remains focused on the discomfort. Especially the evaluation and the subsequent desire for correction must be postponed until later. You should of course notice and pay attention to the resistances that arise, but postpone them until later and possibly focus on them as a separate question.

Be patient with yourself. During the process, stay with your attention inside your body, listen to yourself, wait for what comes up.

Listen to yourself
Listen inside yourself

This exercise has the effect that an unpleasant feeling or pain can approach and be experienced neutrally or even positively. It no longer has to fight for attention with all its might – and in the best case can leave. This power is released and benefits your vitality.

Exercise 11: Body Responses

Nothing is so bad that it does not have something good ... Pain sometimes has a good purpose. They point to too much or too little, they bring an advantage or point to a task which needs to be solved. For example, they indicate too much work – too few breaks – too little exercise, etc. Or are there perhaps sources of conflict and stress which are urging to be solved?

The good cause

If the pain can be questioned directly, it can reveal its meaning.

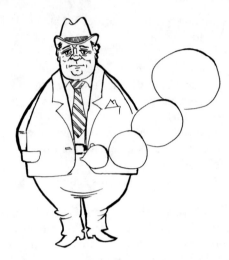

The term *voice* in the following does not only mean something audible. It is often rather an inner image, an intuition or a deep thought.

Implementation   At the beginning and after the end of the exercise, the current pain level on the pain scale is assessed.
- "I now turn my attention into my body […], to my pain spot […] and breathe exactly there […]. Can I put a hand gently on the painful spot?
- What should I be aware of, what should I protect myself from […]?

The voice of pain
- Now I imagine that the pain area has a voice – what would it say to me […]? I give myself enough time to perceive its voice […].
- If there were an emotion attached to this pain, what would it be […]?
- If a movement […], an action or activity were linked to this pain […], what would it look like? What should I do in the future […]? And what should I refrain from doing […]?
- What does the pain tell me – does it still want me to know anything […]? Is there anything else that is missing […]?
- If the problem/pain was already somewhat solved, how would that feel in my body […]?
- I feel for and enjoy this state […].
- I bid you farewell and thank you […]."

What would you answer?

If listening to the inner voice is still difficult, try a "role change": In this, you do not question the pain site like a "foreign person", but slip into the role of the pain, so to speak. How would you answer in the role of the pain now?

Exercise 12: Feeling Behind the Pain

This exercise requires a high degree of openness to one's inner self. The idea is that pain and some activities can be used to avoid something even more unpleasant. Feelings of fear, overwhelm, isolation, boredom, helplessness, anger, and deep sadness sometimes seek a mask to avoid being experienced.

Is something even more unpleasant to be avoided?

Implementation   At the beginning and end of the exercise, rate the current level of pain on a scale of 0–10, keeping hand contact with the pain site if possible.

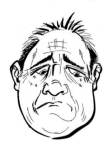

- "I focus my attention on the inside of my body: I feel into my abdomen and chest […]. When I perceive my pain experience, everything I know about my pain, what sensations come to mind […]? Where do unpleasant sensations […] arise? What fears […], worries […], sadness […], anger […], disappointment […] or […] can I recognize […]?"
- "I notice them each as kindly as possible and ask them if it is good to stay with them for a while […]. If so, I stay with each one of you for a while […].
- If the pain with its inconveniences were suddenly magically gone – as if a miracle had happened, all pain gone […] – how would that feel physically […]? What would I then be confronted with, what problems would remain – how would that feel […]? In my job […], in my partnership […], in my family […], in my circle of friends […], in the field of … […]? […]?
- I perceive every arising bodily sensation kindly […] and patiently […].

What if the pain went away?

- I now gently put each body feeling aside and find a suitable place where it can feel at ease […].

Find a good place

- If necessary, I will deal with it in more detail later (you should keep this promise then!).
- I thank you for the knowledge and insights […] and say goodbye to all the pain and feelings with the certainty of knowing they are in good hands […].
- I enjoy and experience for another moment how it would feel if everything was already a bit more relaxed […].
- Then I'll say goodbye slowly …"

In this exercise, an inner distance – taking a few steps back internally – is particularly important in order not to be overwhelmed by emotions.

> ❯ If your emotions regularly become so great that they seem unmanageable, please do not be afraid to ask your doctor or therapist for help.

Rest and Relaxation Techniques

Relaxation has a positive effect – especially on pain

In the midst of experiencing pain, when all the muscles tense, the breath stops, one can hardly imagine being able to relax in a controlled way. But especially in the experience of pain, the positive influence of relaxation techniques is scientifically well proven.

Pain is a stress factor

On the one hand, pain acts as a stressor – causing tension of all kinds, which in turn perpetuates psychophysical dysfunction in the body, so that de-stressing can break this cycle.

Stress increases the sensitivity to pain

On the other hand, (permanent) stress from the (also: former) living environment is a classic pain trigger and amplifier and increases the sensitivity to pain. Emotions such as suffering, fears, anger, excitement – which often go hand in hand with the experience of pain – cause, among other things, an increase in tension in the musculature and vegetative system – even if one does not consciously feel them.

Relaxation reduces anxiety and stress and is incompatible with them, because relaxation is the opposite of stress and tension.

Relaxation is the release of a tense state, it is a pleasant physical and mental feeling of rest and recuperation – a mental break and a phase of regeneration of important bodily functions.

Relaxation means regeneration

It is attainable through inner letting go as well as through exercise and physical effort.

Relaxation has to be practiced and trained, just like you train muscles to be stronger and more enduring. Well practiced, relaxation can then also be used successfully in real stress situations.

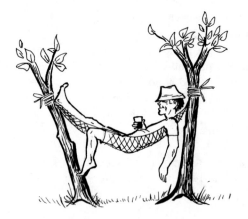

The amazing thing is that after a certain daily practice time (after about 4–6 weeks, sometimes even earlier) you only need to *think about* the relaxation effect to reactively feel relaxation.

The goal is to use relaxation at the first sign of pain and let it take effect so that the pain level can be kept low immediately, loosely based on the motto, "Resist the beginnings!"

The same applies to pain: nip it in the bud

Simple and easy to learn relaxation techniques include:
- Progressive Muscle Relaxation according to Jacobson (PME),
- concentrative relaxation such as Autogenic Training according to Schultz,
- Mindfulness and body awareness exercises,
- Breathing techniques,
- Visualizations such as imagination exercises and fantasy journeys,
- body-oriented methods such as Yoga, Feldenkrais, Alexander Technique, etc.

Practical Tip

Usually, relaxation methods can be used well as self-exercises. For some people it is more motivating to learn and do the exercises in a group with other people. This can happen in courses of the health insurance companies or with psychologists, please inform yourself in each case there.

The Effects of Relaxation Techniques

Relaxation procedures serve to regulate increased arousal and tension. The aim is to achieve a balance to stress and straining tension, in the long term to achieve an appropriate "normal tension".

Relaxation techniques have an effect on both the physical (muscular-vegetative) and psychological level (thoughts, general feelings of hecticness and excitement, moods) and reinforce each other: calmness and composure require a relaxed body sensation – and vice versa. Stress and pain subside, and well-being and performance are increased.

Relaxation works on a physical and psychological level …

But relaxation can do even more: it also helps to reduce anxiety, to gain strength, to take up activities and to initiate changes.

… and helps to initiate changes

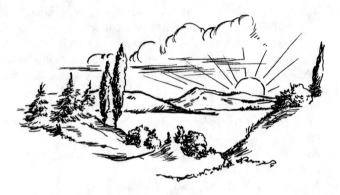

The individual effects of relaxation:

Balance
— Inner peace and balance are promoted.

— Muscle relaxation regulates the blood flow in the body. Tense muscles, on the other hand, prevent an optimal blood and oxygen supply – both to the muscles themselves and to the other organs.

Breathe
— Breathing regulates itself, influencing the depth, rhythm and space of breathing as well as the breathing movement. Stress and pain always have an effect on breathing: It becomes shallower, more hectic and inefficient.

Body Awareness
— The body awareness is strengthened. By sensitizing body perception, signs of stress, tension and pain are noticed much earlier, thus creating the possibility of countermeasures.

Vascular system
— The vascular system is positively influenced, the vegetative nervous system (responsible for blood pressure, digestion, sweating etc.) is regulated.

Pain tolerance
— The pain threshold is raised, the pain tolerance is increased. One actually feels less pain.

What to Consider in Practical Application

It does not work without practice

Learning relaxation techniques is similar to learning and automating other skills (like riding a bike, playing an instrument, etc.). It is a learning process, it takes practice, concentration and commitment. Finally, it succeeds without effort and is almost automatic.

But even if you have long since mastered the relaxation exercises, it is necessary to use them again and again, just as a muscle must continue to be exercised in order to remain functional. Unfortunately, many people stop practicing after the first feelings of success, because it no longer seems necessary to them.

Even remembering to relax can help

The success can be felt very quickly, at the latest after 2–4 weeks. And after a few weeks of practice, simply remembering the experienced state of relaxation is enough to release tension and pain.

Initially, you should choose the timing of your relaxation exercise according to your pain level, meaning you exercise when the pain is *not too extreme.*

In the first 6 weeks you should practice at least 2 times a day, better 3 times, for 20 min each. Later, 1–2 times a day is enough – and of course as needed.

At the beginning it may not be easy to concentrate on yourself for 20 min, sounds and sensations are distracting at first. Not every relaxation succeeds immediately or always equally well. This is normal and the same applies to all other activities. The more composed you can be about the situation, the sooner relaxation will be possible.

Be patient with yourself

A quiet environment is also important at the beginning, so that you can really be undisturbed and without internal time pressure. The chosen time of day is basically irrelevant. It is best to incorporate the practice time into the daily routine in such a way that it is automatically remembered (e.g. practice *always* after lunch, before going to sleep, etc.). Habituation then occurs more quickly.

You can literally counter-condition your body over time when signs of tension or negative feelings arise. As soon as your body reacts to certain trigger situations, e.g. with fear or tension, you can also get it to respond to this stress with relaxation. The principle is very simple, but enormously effective: If a certain disturbing affect occurs, you counteract it with relaxation training. The more often you repeat this process, the more the organism gets used to reacting in this way.

Immediately respond with relaxation

It makes sense to first practice relaxation thoroughly in senso, i.e. mentally, and later it can be applied directly in real stress/tension situations so that the level of pain and negative feelings can be kept low.

Exercise: Initiation of Relaxation

You can place the introductory module described here at the beginning of any procedure discussed in subsequent chapters.

Module: Relaxation Initiation

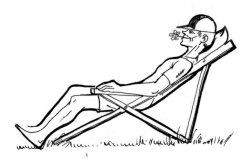

You can speak these instructions on a recording device, but you can also memorize the individual sections and then go through them mentally.

Comfortable body position

1. Now take time and rest to relax. Find a suitable, relaxed position. The eyes can be closed, or – if that is considered uncomfortable – the gaze is set to "far away".

Determination of the pain level

2. Visualize your stress or pain scale and assess your level of tension or pain between 0 and 10.

Body perception

3. Be aware of your body in a concentrated way. Feel the support surface, the contact areas with the support and the body parts in between. Go through the different parts of your body like a scanner and feel their state of tension.

Breathe

4. Feel your breathing:
   - the *path* that the breath takes from the nose to the deep abdomen,
   - the *movements* that the body makes with each inhalation and exhalation,
   - the *directions* in which the breath flows,
   - the *breathing rhythm* and the *breathing* pauses.
   - Experience how oxygen is taken in with every *inhalation*, and consumed and tension is released with every *exhalation* […].

Practical Tip

Combination with a signal word

Relaxation exercises become even more efficient when they are combined with breathing and a signal word (that suits you!). For example, with each *exhalation* you say or think of a term such as *calm, relaxed, unconcerned, relieved* – and experience this state as intensively as possible.

Include sensory perceptions

The more consciously one feels the tension and relaxation and includes all current sensory perceptions (what do I see – smell – taste – hear – feel right now?), the deeper the relaxation and the more pleasant the mood will become.

Enjoy the idea of rest, relaxation, and that there is nothing more important to do right now.

Disturbing thoughts?

Practical Tip

It is normal to notice wandering thoughts, disturbing bodily sensations or sounds. Notice them, let them go again, and continue practicing. For very persistent thoughts, you can use helpful images (imaginings), such as imagining clouds or train cars pulling the thoughts away with you. Or you can organize your troublesome thoughts, imaginarily "sorting" them into little boxes or shelves with the promise: "Not now! But later." And then find time for the problem!

Progressive Muscle Relaxation (PMR) according to E. Jacobson

PMR is a self-relaxation method that was developed in the 1930s by the American Edmund Jacobson. The technique is easy to learn, scientifically very well researched and can be excellently applied in everyday practice. Muscular tensions, vegetative and central nervous excitations (such as restlessness, sweating, palpitations, pain) are reduced, one feels altogether calmer, calmer and fresher.

Self-relaxation

In addition to the sensation of relaxation, it is also about the restoration of the so-called *muscle sense,* the ability to use one's muscle power economically and sensibly again. With increasing practice, it becomes possible to sense exactly where too much, inappropriate or permanent tension is being exerted.

Muscle Sense

For this purpose, some essential muscle groups are first tensed for 7–10 seconds and then loosened, while at the same time paying very concentrated attention to the onset of sensations that are felt in the muscles.

Depending on your needs, either rather powerful contractions or only a minimally noticeable tension are preferred, in case of high painfulness even a mentally imagined tension is sufficient! Try out what is good for you, the best measure must be found individually. However, cramping or increased pain should not occur under any circumstances.

Try out what is good for you

Also make sure that breathing continues to flow rhythmically, press breathing should be avoided.

After releasing the tension, it is important to feel the relaxation – or better: the difference between tension and relaxation – for about 30 more seconds and to enjoy this.

Difference between tension and relaxation

Application Tips for PMR

Relaxation initiation

— Again, you can speak the entire instruction on a recorder or memorize individual sections of the exercise and then mentally play through them.

— It may be useful to *initiate relaxation* before performing the exercise (section "Initiation of Relaxation").

— During the exercise you can sit or lie down, whichever seems more comfortable. Later, when you are more practiced, you can relax in all positions, in all situations.

— The tension of the mentioned muscle regions should be held for 7–10 seconds each and consciously perceived. Then release the tension again, slowly and consciously.

— Please make sure that only the specified muscles are tensed and not – in the course of a chain reaction – other parts of the body.

— After the exercise you should feel and let the relaxation happen for about 30 seconds. Consciously notice the difference between tension and relaxation.

Exercise 13: Progressive Muscle Relaxation: Long Form

Long form: All muscle groups are tightened individually

If you are not yet familiar with progressive muscle relaxation, it is best to practice the long form first. This involves first tensing and then relaxing all muscle groups individually: the hands and arms, the face, the neck and shoulders, the torso, both legs and the buttocks.

Later, when you are more practiced, you can choose the short form, which is faster to perform.

Implementation   At the beginning and end of the exercise, rate the instantaneous pain level on a scale of 0–10.

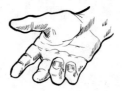

- **Hands and Arms**

1. Clench your **right hand** into a fist, feeling the tension up into your forearm as consciously as possible – then slowly release and relax – feeling the difference between tension and relaxation – repeat this process again.
2. Bend the **right elbow** (tense the biceps muscle), observe the tension – relax – feel the difference … – repeat once.
3. Clench your **left hand** into a fist, feel the tension up into your forearm – release – feel the difference – repeat once.
4. Bend the **left elbow**, feel the tension – relax – feel the difference – repeat once.
5. Extend **both arms** and press firmly against the surface (activate the triceps muscles) – notice the tension – release – feel the difference – repeat once.

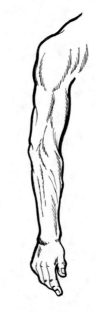

- **Face**

1. Wrinkle or fold your **forehead** – notice this tension carefully – then slowly release and relax again – consciously feel the difference – repeat this process once.
2. Pull the **Eyebrows** together – notice tension – release – feel the difference – repeat once.
3. Squint your **eyes** – notice the tension – release – feel the difference – repeat once.
4. Wrinkle **nose** – notice tension – release – feel the difference – repeat once.
5. Press **lips** together or pucker them ("kissing mouth") – perceive tension – release – feel the difference – repeat once.
6. Gently (!) clench your **teeth**, tense the jaw muscles – notice the feeling of tension – release – feel – repeat once.
7. Press the **tongue** against the palate – notice the feeling of tension – release – feel the difference – repeat once.
8. Close your eyes, move your eyeballs far to the right, hold your gaze there for a while and perceive the tension – move back to the centre and feel the relaxation – then move your gaze to the left – hold your gaze and feel the tension – release – trace. Then the same procedure with the gaze upwards – downwards and also diagonally in all directions. Hold the tension in each case and feel – release – trace.

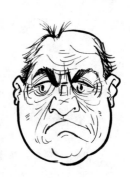

■   **Neck and Shoulders**

Neck

1. Press your **head** *backwards* into/against the pad – feel the tension in the neck muscles – release and relax again – feel the difference between tension and relaxation – repeat once.
2. Slowly *turn the* head to the *right*, as if against resistance – notice the feeling of tension – release – feel the difference – repeat once. Then *turn the* head to the *left in the* same way – perceive the feeling of tension – release – feel the difference – repeat once.

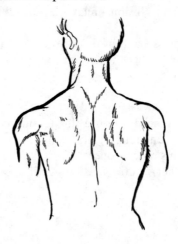

3. *Bend* the head *forward* (pull the chin towards the breastbone) – notice the feeling of tension – release – feel – repeat once.

Shoulders

4. *Pull up the* **shoulders** towards the ears – notice the feeling of tension – release – feel the difference – repeat once.
5. Bring shoulders *together in front* – feel the tension – release the tension – feel the difference – repeat once.
6. Pull the shoulder blades *backwards* (towards the spine) – notice the feeling of tension – release – feel – repeat once.

■   **Hull**

Back muscles

1. Now tense your **back muscles** by going into a slight hollow back (when lying down this means that only the buttocks and shoulders are resting) – notice the feeling of tension carefully – then release the tension – feel the difference – repeat once.

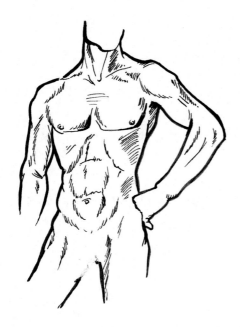

Abdominal muscles   2.   Tense the abdominal muscles (as if you wanted to ward off a light blow to the abdomen) – perceive the feeling of tension – release – trace – repeat once.

- **Buttocks and Legs**
1. Tense your **right half of the buttocks** and feel the tension up into your thigh – release the tension again – and consciously notice the difference between tightening and relaxing – repeat this process once.
2. Tense the **left half of the buttocks**, feel the tension up into the thigh – release – trace – repeat once.
3. Press **both thighs** together – perceive tension – release – trace – repeat once.
4. Tense the **right calf**, pull the right foot up towards the head and at the same time press the calf into the pad – notice the feeling of tension – release – feel – repeat once.
5.   Tense the **left calf**, pull the left foot up towards the head and at the same time press the calf into the pad – notice the feeling of tension – release – feel – repeat once.
6. Curl (grasp) all **toes** – perceive feeling of tension – release – trace – repeat once.

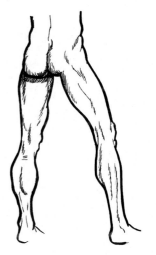

Afterwards, feel all parts of the body again in a relaxed state. Where residual tension is registered, you can repeat the tension/relaxation cycle.

Tracing

Then enjoy the relaxed state for 2–3 min …

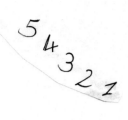

■ **Withdrawal: Ending the Relaxation**
1. Set yourself up internally for quitting.
2. With your eyes closed, count backwards from 5 to 1.
3. Tighten both arms, loll, stretch and straighten.
4. Breathe in deeply, exhale forcefully – and then open your eyes.

Of course, the withdrawal is unnecessary if the PMR is used as a sleep aid.

Exercise 14: Progressive Muscle Relaxation: Short Form

Short relaxation

When body relaxation is reliably achieved with the help of the long form – usually after 2–4 weeks of regular daily practice – you can move on to the short form.

This is divided into two phases, first the **whole body** is tensed at once, then **four muscle groups** are contracted in succession, in the following order:
1. Hands – arms,
2. Face – Neck,
3. Shoulder – trunk,
4. Buttocks – legs.

Implementation   At the beginning and end of the exercise, rate the instantaneous pain level on a scale of 0–10.

■ **Phase 1: Whole Body Tension**

Synchronous relaxation of
the whole body

Get into a sitting position that is comfortable for you or into the side position.

Then roll your entire body in the following manner:

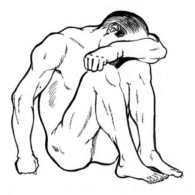

1. The back is bent as if you wanted to make a cat's hump, please pull in the head, put the chin on the chest,
2. both arms are crossed in front of the chest,

3. then pull your shoulders up towards your ears,
4. afterwards tense the abdomen and buttocks,
5. while pulling the legs,
6. last tense all the muscles of the face, pressing the tongue against the palate.

All muscle groups should then be tensed simultaneously – together – and held for 7–10 s. During this time, make sure your breathing is calm. Be as aware as possible of the tension. Then release the tension – and feel the difference for about 30 s. Repeat this once or twice.

This is followed in the same way by the contraction and relaxation of the following four individual muscle groups.

■ **Phase 2: Four Muscle Groups**

Remain in your chosen sitting or lying position. In the following, tense whole muscle groups one after the other and hold the tension for 7–10 s at a time and consciously perceive it. Continue to breathe calmly.

Four muscle groups

Then slowly or, depending on your preference, suddenly release the tension – and consciously feel the difference for about 30 s. Repeat this process 2–3 times.

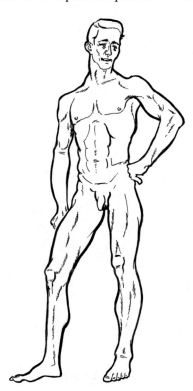

Order

Work in this order:

1. **Arms**: Simultaneously tense both arms by bending them with clenched fists – perceive hold and tension – then release and feel the difference in tension.
2. **Face**: Simultaneously frown, squint both eyes, wrinkle the nose, press the lips together, slightly clench the teeth and pull the head in – notice the tension – release it again – feel the difference.
3. **Torso**: Simultaneously pull the shoulders back towards the spine, tense the back muscles and at the same time go into a slight hollow back, counter-tension the abdomen as if you wanted to ward off a light blow – perceive the tension – release it – and feel it.
4. **Legs**: Simultaneously tense buttocks, thighs and calves, pull feet up towards the head and let all toes grip – perceive tension – release – feel.

At the end you can once again feel the entire body in its relaxation – and enjoy it for a while …

PMR can also be performed in everyday stressful situations

If PMR has already been practiced extensively and works well, it can be used directly in your everyday environment – with time you will even master its use in the middle of stressful situations. It is then sufficient to tense all four muscle groups of the arms, face, trunk and leg muscles at the same time (if you want it to be inconspicuous, of course, without the face muscles). Again, hold for 7–10 seconds and feel tension – slowly release and notice the difference in tension for 30 seconds. The exercise can be repeated as needed.

Practical Tip

Signal word

If you have learned to couple a signal word to the relaxation exercises at the same time, such as "Relaxation!", "Take it easy!" or whatever else you like, and this signal word – similar to a mantra – is continuously repeated during the relaxation exercise, then after a while this word alone will be sufficient – without prior tensioning of the muscles – to achieve effective relaxation! Just as sometimes your mouth automatically waters when you just think of lemons …

Relaxation short forms are very practical in everyday situations that require a short, unobtrusive relaxation, for example:
- after anger situations to cool down (e.g. in traffic),
- in waiting situation to use time wisely,
- when, due to a lack of time, relaxation has to be reduced to short break times.

An important goal of PME is the re-learning of the *muscle sense* mentioned earlier. Ideally, progressive muscle relaxation makes it possible to feel again in every situation where muscles are tensing too much, too uneconomically, and a very specific relaxation of these muscles is learned. While in the beginning the whole PMR-exercises are needed, later a conscious sensing of existing muscle tension is sufficient; the relaxation then happens by simply remembering (!) the feeling of relaxation.

Exercise 15: Concentrative Relaxation

If there is sufficient experience with progressive muscle relaxation, relaxation can therefore finally also be achieved through concentration, i.e. through mental control.

Mental attention

> The best-known method of concentrative relaxation is Autogenic Training. However, learning it requires a high level of discipline and must be well implemented. This method should therefore be acquired under guidance, e.g. in special courses. Otherwise, the dropout rate is very high – and so is the disappointment.

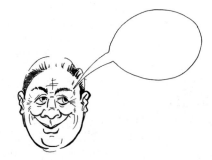

Just the concentrative, conscious turning to a body region can relax the tissue there, increase the blood circulation and harmonize the vegetative system. This has an overall strengthening and pain-relieving effect.

In the following, a *tension check* is presented, which is very well applicable in everyday situations, feasible in front of the TV, during breaks or on the road. Here, too, practicing several times a day is the quickest way to success.

Voltage check

Implementation   At the beginning and end of the exercise, rate the instantaneous pain level on a scale of 0–10.

Let the attention wander
from the head to the toes

Find a position that suits you and loosen your body [...].

Now mentally experience (in your mind) a situation that is pleasant for you [...]. After a while, go through your body with your attention in slow motion, "slice by slice" from head to toes [...]. Do this really slowly and consciously, so that you could stop at any second. As you do this, feel for the places where there are signs of tension/pain or other interference fields such as itching, a feeling of pressure ... [...]. In this way you can also determine where there are "unloved" places or body regions. To integrate these again is especially important!

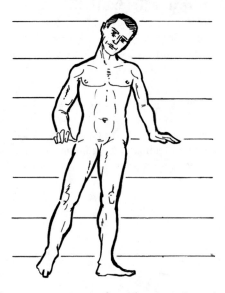

Dwell on the point of
tension

Focus on one area of tension at a time, dwell there – and:

1. Breathe very specifically there. The inhalation should hit the pain/tension area as precisely as possible.
2. Then with each exhalation, virtually push or squeeze the pain away as if to bring it out of your body.
3. If any remnants of tension remain at this point, linger a moment with your attention. Welcome it as readily as possible, then "invite it out" with a friendly attitude. Then imagine the tension escaping with each exhalation.

Replace with a pleasant
feeling

4. then send/put a pleasant body feeling to the previously tense place: e.g. warmth, strength, a touch etc.. ... Just what would be good for you now.

Then choose the next tense, painful area of the body and repeat the exercise.

Finally, linger for 2–3 min and feel inside your body.

Exercise 16: Relaxation through Tapping Acupressure

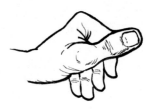

In this section, the focus is on the pain with its physical and emotional accompaniments, while at the same time pressing, tapping or rubbing certain points (acupuncture points) on the body with one of your thumbs.

This technique can cause an altered neuronal connection in the CNS, which gives room to new experiences regarding pain and emotions and thus enables pain relearning. In addition, an intense revival of pain perception occurs in a controlled, i.e. "harmless" situation; relaxation or pain relief follows reactively.

Altered neuronal connection

Instead of pain, stress symptoms or distressing feelings can also be treated in this way.

Implementation   To begin with, rate the discomfort/pain you are feeling right now on a scale you have imagined. Which number between 0 and 10 (0 as no pain, 10 as unbearable pain) best corresponds to the pain you feel now?

■ **Step 1**

Now consciously perceive the pain and describe it as precisely as possible: try to find a name, a heading or a characteristic that best describes the quality of your current pain.

Perceive and name

■■ **Example**
"A sharp, searing pain that has annoyed me for the last hour and made me very angry."

Try to feel this sensation as intensely as possible for 1–2 min.

■ **Step 2**
Find a balancing formula (or an affirmation, Exercise 6) or something that expresses relaxation for you and would be especially good for you.

Compensation formula

■■ **Examples**
"I know the pain will go away in a moment." "I look forward to …" "Though this pain angers me, I accept it …"

Or think, for example, of the heating pad on the back of your neck that would do you good now; or experience the anticipation of a cup of tea; or could you enjoy the beautiful surroundings in this situation?

Again, experience this pleasant sensation/balancing formula as intensely as possible for 1–2 min, and say it – even with exaggerated emphasis, inwardly or audibly.

■ **Step 3**

Find acupuncture point

In addition, find an acupuncture point, it is located between the collarbone and the shoulder joint. Palpate your collarbone, then move to the upper part of the collarbone towards the shoulder joint. The acupuncture point is located just before the shoulder joint at the junction with the pectoral muscle. It is more sensitive than its surroundings, yet it can be treated quite forcefully.

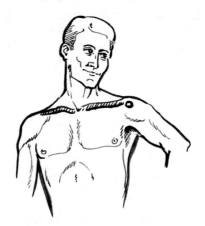

This point should be pressed, tapped or rubbed with one of your thumbs throughout the process!

■■ **Alternative**

Use the four fingertips of the dominant hand (usually on the right) to tap or rub the outer edge of the other hand.

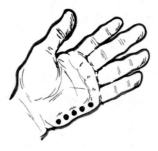

Alternating pain perception and affirmation

Step 1 and step 2 are combined alternately – so first feel the problem inwardly as actively and intensely as possible and then your situation or affirmation that you feel is pleasant. To reinforce this, you can say it inwardly or audibly out loud.

Meanwhile, hold or tap your chosen pressure point the entire time.

■ **Practice Completion**

This is followed by another rating of the pain perceived right now on the scale of 0–10. What has changed?

The pain should have decreased by at least two scale points. Otherwise, you can repeat this process until the pain is significantly reduced or, at best, dropped to zero.

Pain reduction by at least 2 scale points

If no success is noticeable, perhaps a modified compensatory formula or affirmation should be found. This should really suit you, otherwise inner resistance will arise. One possibility to prevent resistance would be a limited approval of the intension.

Resistors

■■ **Example**

"Even though I don't believe in it at the moment, I feel … and look forward to …"

After some practice, you can choose a short form for steps 1 and 2.

Short form

■■ **Example**

"Even though I still have this pain, I'm looking forward to …"

Or even shorter, "This remaining pain – and I look forward to …"

Exercise 17: Relaxation Through Eye Movements

Here, too, a situation that is perceived as unpleasant, anxiety- or pain-inducing is intensively reanimated and then processed.

Implementation Take a rating of your pain on the scale of 0–10 before and after each exercise process.

1. Be aware of your pain or imagine the problematic situation mentally and emotionally as intensely as possible. Look on an inner screen, so to speak: What exactly do I see […], hear […], smell […], feel […]?

   Intensive experience

2. Pause in this situation for 1–2 min and be as aware of it as possible.

3. Now follow for about 30 s strong eyeball movements very far to the right and left to the corners of the eyes – in rapid alternation. Alternatively, the eyes can also be rolled in a circle.

   Oscillating eye movements

4. Then bring to mind a situation or sensation that you have experienced as pleasant – it can be remembered or constructed in your imagination: What feels good now, what would feel good? Perceive this with all your senses.

5. Now again quickly and forcefully move both eyes alternately to the left and right.
6. After about a minute you should trace ...: How does it feel now [...]? What has changed?

This technique can bring about an altered neural connection in the CNS that makes room for new experiences and pain relearning.

It requires little effort, is easy to try out and can be integrated very well into everyday life.

Exercise 18: Relaxation Through Pain Tolerance

This technique is a must for people in pain!

It releases physical tension, harmonizes important acupuncture points (of the bladder meridian) and increases pain tolerance. This means that not only muscular tensions are reduced, but that the entire "pain reporting centre" is trained so that it is activated much later. Pain hypersensitivity and consequently anticipatory anxiety decrease noticeably.

What you need as a tool is only a tennis ball, which is divided into two equal halves. Then for advanced players are suitable two whole tennis balls.

Implementation   The exercise is best done lying on your back, but it is also possible to do it standing in front of a wall. Assume a position that is as comfortable as possible.

Before and after the exercise process, take a rating of your pain on the scale of 0–10.

Body awareness

1. A relaxation exercise would be a good way to start. If this is impractical, a short body awareness of the points of contact between body and support is sufficient.

Pressure points and breath control

2. Now place the two tennis balls or halves symmetrically on the right and left under the buttocks and gently lower yourself down on them. Stay like this for at least 90 s and breathe into the painful areas.
3. Then push the tennis balls further up the lowest part of the spine, symmetrically each right and left, as close together as possible. Again, you should maintain this position for 90 s and consciously breathe there.
4. Successively put the balls a few centimeters higher, hold each for at least one and a half minutes and breathe there until you reach the cervical spine. Of course, you may also work on other painful areas, e.g. in the shoulder girdle or lumbar region.

Once you have learned to accept the pain (and the tennis balls really can't break anything!), this acupressure causes both a release of pain and tension and an increase in tolerance.

Accept pain

> ❯ Initially, you may feel sore muscles in the first few days, but this usually goes away after 3–5 days. Once this phase is overcome, you will no longer want to do without this exercise.

Relaxation Through Body Awareness and Sensory Perception

The training of body mindfulness and sensory perception has been of great importance in pain therapy for some time. From a neurophysiological point of view, mindful perception can even directly inhibit the "emotional system". That means: In a phase of mindfulness, pain can hardly be felt at the same time.

High priority

Conscious concentration, especially on something pleasant, not only steers away from stressful thoughts and pain, it also has an overall balancing, relaxing and restorative effect.

By feeling your own body you also gain the ability to become familiar with your body and to feel at home in it (again). It is then easier to accept your body and not to perceive it exclusively in a worrying, dismissive way; body awareness and self-confidence are mutually dependent.

Becoming familiar with your own body

Normally our attention is directed outwards. Conscious sensing as inner perception of the body, mindfulness of thoughts, feelings and sensory perceptions often have to be rediscovered.

In all concentration exercises it is important to *experience* the immediate present state of mind, i.e. not to remember only mentally.

Experience condition

Attention is focused in such a way that at this moment nothing seems more important than the very moment of perception.

Exercise 19: Body Walk

Here the whole body is perceived mindfully, all arising sensations – without rejecting them – are welcomed. If the sensations, the experience, feel rather unpleasant, then this can also be noted mindfully.

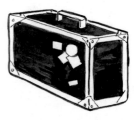

Implementation   Before and after the exercise process, take a rating of your pain on the scale of 0–10.

Relaxation initiation   It is best to start with a relaxation induction (section "Induction of Relaxation").

Right arm
1. Now concentrate your thoughts on the right hand – try to feel the right thumb – the index finger – the middle finger – the ring finger – the little finger – and dwell there each time […].
2. Then direct your attention to the back of the hand – the forearm – the elbow – and linger for some time in each case […]. Continue breathing calmly and regularly […].
3. Move on to the right upper arm – to the right shoulder – along the collarbone inwards to the breastbone – and dwell there […].

Left arm
4. Direct the draw attention along the left collarbone into the left shoulder – linger wherever it is comfortable […].
5. Then wander downwards into the left upper arm – the forearm – to the back of the hand […]. Concentrate your attention on the individual fingers one after the other […]. The whole rest of the body remains calm and relaxed […].

Body center
6. Focus your attention on the centre of the body – there the abdominal wall rises and falls in rhythm with the breath […]. In the depth you feel the warmth of the abdominal cavity […].

Legs
7. Then go downward into the right leg: the thigh – the lower leg – the foot –, and linger in each case as long as you like […].
8. Then pay attention to the left foot – to the left calf – the knee – the thigh – the left groin […].

Back to the center of the body
9. Then return to the center of the body. Feel for it: Does warmth – heaviness – lightness – a tingling – … make itself felt somewhere […]?
10. Now gradually finish this exercise – loll and stretch extensively – breathe deeply a few times – now open your eyes – and then slowly straighten up.

Feel for it: How does your whole body feel now […]?

Exercise 20: The Good Place

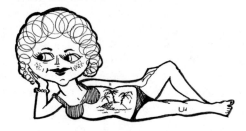

Again, it is best to start with an introduction to relaxation (section "Introduction of Relaxation").

Relaxation initiation

Take a rating of your pain on the scale of 0–10 before and after the exercise.

1. Now feel attentively into your body. Calmly move from the feet upwards over the interior of the torso to the head, and gently and benevolently look for a place that feels good right now […].

Find a pleasant body part

2. Focus your attention on this pleasant spot for a moment and let the body sensation take effect […].
3. Try to describe the pleasant sensation somehow: It feels warm, safe, light […].

Describe sensation

4. Linger with your attention in this place and ask yourself: What is the best, the most pleasant thing about this place […]?
5. Feel the emerging sensation, still stay with it without having to change anything – and enjoy it […]. Then feel whether this positive sensation can spread a little, perhaps to neighbouring regions […].
6. Now gradually finish this exercise – loll and stretch extensively – breathe deeply a few times – now open your eyes – and then slowly straighten up […].

Feel for it: How does your whole body feel now […]?

Exercise 21: Sensory Channels

We perceive the world through the various sensory channels: Informations and interpretations reach the organism through sight, hearing, smell, taste, touch, movement and bodily sensation.

Most people prefer to use 1–2 different channels.

Expansion of the sensory perceptions

The reduction to one or a few sensory perceptions, however, filters out others; we then perceive in a limited and one-sided way. An expansion of the possibilities of perception makes us more flexible, enriches our experience and distracts us from painful sensations.

Which sensory type are you?

Pay attention to which sensory type you are: Through which channel do you take in your environment and your inner world? Which sensations seem clear and easy to remember, and to which channels do you have little connection?

- **Visual Sense**

Eye

Do you perceive your environment mainly by sight, i.e. taking it in with your eyes, forming an inner picture?

- **Auditory Sense**

Ear

Do you perceive by hearing and listening, do you remember well what you have heard, do you listen to your inner voice?

- **Sense of Smell**

Nose

Do you become aware of smells, are you reminded by smells?

- **Sense of Taste**

Tongue

Do you enjoy absorbing and savoring flavors?

- **Kinesthetic Sense**

Body awareness

What do you feel? Do you have a good body feeling for posture and movement, do you experience strong physical feelings of well-being or discomfort?

If you want to expand your sensory perceptions, you should consciously use the channels that are rather weak in you.

Implementation Everywhere, in all activities, you can consciously perceive your surroundings. The most practical way to do this is in normal everyday life, for example, on the way to work, while waiting, on a trip, during a professional activity, and so on.

The following small exercises – which can also be carried out imaginarily, i.e. in the inner imagination – help with this training:

- **Visual Sense**

"I look around carefully: What is there to see in my surroundings? What does everything look like exactly: the individual shapes, the colours, the sizes, the surfaces?

What is the most beautiful thing about it for me?"

- **Auditory Sense**

"What sounds, tones, voices do I perceive? What does … sound like in my imagination? What does it remind me of?
What do I like about it?"

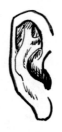

- **Sense of Smell**

"I perceive the scent of …. What does … smell like in my memory? What does it remind me of? What do i feel about it?"

- **Sense of Taste**

Taste of … melting exactly on the tongue – "What can I perceive? What does it remind me of?"

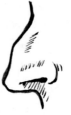

- **Touch**

"I consciously touch and feel things in my environment – how do the different materials feel? How do I recognize them, how are they different? What do they remind me of?"

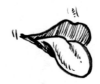

- **Kinesthetic Sense**

"How does … affect me – does it trigger a pleasant or rather an uncomfortable feeling in me? What mood do I feel, how do I feel about …? What touches me?"

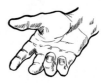

Exercise 22: The Apple

In the following exercise, all sensory channels are addressed while you perceive an apple more closely.

Implementation Before and after the exercise, determine the value of your pain on the scale of 0–10.

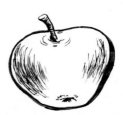

Grasp with all senses

Place an apple about 50 cm away in front of you. Position it so that you can look at it closely. Your task is now to grasp the apple with as many senses as possible.

1. Concentrate and look at the outside of the apple first: How big is it? What shape is it? What is its skin like? What colors do you notice? Are there any distinctive features such as spots, dents, or punctures? […]
2. Then close your eyes and take the apple in your hand. Feel its weight, weigh it lightly. Feel the surface and shape, and feel how the skin yields softly despite a strong touch. Hold the apple against a cheek – how cool and smooth the skin is! Bring it to your lips and touch it. […]
3. Can you smell the fresh, sweet scent? Now take a bite of the apple: how does it taste, what does the taste remind you of? […]

4. What is the sound of biting into the apple and chewing?
5. How is the sensation in the mouth? How do you like it? […]

Then put the apple back and repeat all the impressions again with your eyes closed. What *particularly* caught your attention: the bitter taste of a bitten apple core; the pliability of its stem or …?

Gently push aside disturbing thoughts

Practical Tip
If superfluous thoughts come to you during the exercise, gently push them aside for a short while and then refocus on the apple.

Exercise 23: Points of Contact

In this exercise the senses of touch, physical contact and inner perception are particularly addressed. This is an ideal way to redirect attention in the case of pain.

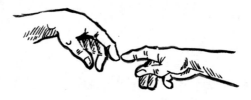

Implementation   Before and after the exercise, determine the value of your pain on the scale of 0–10.

Contact contacts

(D) While sitting for about 2 min, try to perceive the contact between your buttocks and the seat surface […]. "Where is the strongest pressure – how does the rest feel […]? How much of the support surface can be felt – where does it stop […]? Is there a difference between the right and left sides […]? Is this seat comfortable for me […], or what should I change?"

Body, Head

(E) Feel **lying** on your back: "At which points does my body touch the support […]? Where are the heels felt – one heel compared to the other […]? The calves – the buttocks – the sacrum – the back – how many vertebrae lie on the floor […]? The shoulder blades – how do they relate to the spine – how does one shoulder blade relate to the other? The shoulders: How do I feel the distance they are from the floor […]? The head – how do I feel its weight and the point at which it touches the floor [...]? How do I perceive the body support surface as a whole [...]?"

(F) Place both **palms** together, as gently as possible, for about 2 min. "What do I feel [...]? Where are points of contact – where are there gaps [...]? Can I make the touch even softer – without losing contact [...]? And how does stronger/then stronger pressure feel [...]? What do I feel most comfortable with [...]? What would my hands most like to do right now [...]?" | Hands

(G) You feel your **lips** touching for 2 min [...]: "How strong or gentle is the pressure [...]? How would I trace the contours of my lips without a mirror [...]? How little touch is felt just before the mouth opens [...]? How do my lips feel from the inside as my tongue glides along them [...]? How does the tension of my lips change when I smile [...]?" | Lips

Relaxation Through Breathing

Breathing as a partly conscious, partly unconscious physical process is always also a parameter for inner and outer tension. During stress, pain, fear, etc. we breathe differently than in a state of relaxation.

Conversely, breathing can be used to influence the physical and mental tension level. Many body and relaxation methods make use of this knowledge.

Breathing influences many physiological processes in the entire body and of course also in the pain process: Blood circulation and oxygen supply are stimulated, the mobility of the tissue increases, the vegetative nervous system harmonizes – as well as the physical well-being.

Breathing influences the processes in the entire body

Exercise 24: Breath Awareness

Before using special breathing techniques, it is advisable to first become aware of your breathing. Just being mindful often already serves an enormous relaxation and pain relief.

Take your time. Let "it" breathe, don't force a change!

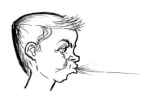

Implementation   Take a rating of your pain on the scale of 0–10 before and after each exercise process.

1. Notice the **path** your breathing takes: How does the breath glide through the nostrils, the root of the nose, the nasopharynx, the trachea, the bronchi, and into the lungs, the abdomen [...]? Observe as closely as possible.

Airway

Breath movements

2. Which areas of your body **move** when you breathe, which more and which less […]? Notice the individual spaces – in the front, back and side direction: Feel the movements, the lifting and lowering of the rib cage, the diaphragm, the lower rib arches, the abdominal cavity up to the pelvic region. Also feel the back, the shoulders in their movement […].

Breathing rhythm

3. Observe the **inhalation** and the **exhalation alternately**: Which phase lasts longer? When are there pauses in breathing? How many breaths (in – out – pause) do you count per minute […]?

Breath quality

4. What is the **quality** of your breath? Do you feel the freshness, the vitality, the lightness that the breath brings […]?

Practical Tip

You can train your breath awareness in everyday life every now and then in between: at home or at work, in the waiting room, at meetings, etc.. Often 3–5 min of practice are enough – for relaxation and as a concentration exercise.

Exercise 25: Special Breathing Techniques

Gentle breath modulation

If breath awareness works well, exercises for gentle (!) breath modulation can be used.

The goal is the most relaxed breathing possible, the characteristics of which are:

- less than 10 breaths per minute at rest,
- a pause for breath between inhalation and exhalation,
- a steady rhythm with a prolonged exhalation phase,
- breathing circular fills especially the abdominal cavity – to the lower abdomen.

The exercises calm, relax, promote concentration and have a pain-reducing effect. Already about 20 gently guided breaths usually relieve or dissolve pain.

The following techniques can be performed as special exercises or integrated into suitable everyday activities. It is not necessary to practice all the individual exercises listed. Pick out the ones that suit you best.

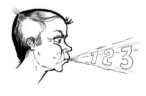

Implementation   At the beginning and end of the exercise, rate the instantaneous pain level on a scale of 0–10.

If possible, choose a comfortable posture in a sitting or supine position, hands placed lightly on the abdomen, feeling the widening and lowering of the torso.

■ **Zilgrei Breathing**
1. You start with a calm inhalation phase through the nose – counting to 3.
2. This is followed by a pause for 3 beats (do not hold your breath or press).
3. The following exhalation is done through the almost closed mouth (lip brake), while counting backwards from 3 to 1.
4. This is followed by a pause for breath, counting to 3 again.

Inhalation 3 time beats, exhalation 3 time beats

So one breathing cycle includes: inhalation – pause – exhalation – pause.

This breathing cycle should be repeated several times. Then feel for it: How does it feel now?

You decide for yourself how long a time beat is. With practice you can increase to 5 or 7 time strokes.

■ **Sigh**
Sigh as loudly as the situation allows, letting yourself fall deeper and deeper inside. Repeat this several times. Yawning has an equally deeply relaxing effect. It can be provoked by rolling your tongue backwards or by imagining that you have a large fruit in your gullet. This relaxes the whole body and especially the muscles in the jaw and neck area.

Sighing and yawning release tension

■ **Contact Breathing**

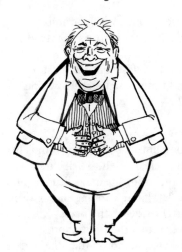

1. First place your hands on the right and left sides of your waist. Then repeat this on the abdomen – or on the lumbar spine – or on the sternum – or on the ribcage. Try out different areas.
2. Gradually increase the pressure of the hands, and breathe into this pressure – as if to "breathe away" the hands.

Increase pressure almightily

3. Repeat several times, afterwards feel without hand contact. What has changed?

■ **Spiral Breathing**

1. In the depth of the abdomen, imagine the beginning of a spiral.

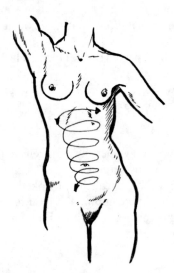

Breathing circles in the abdomen

2. This turns larger and larger circles with the inhalation – and takes the same path back to the starting point with the exhalation.
3. Let the breath "turn" once clockwise, once against.
4. Repeat this process several times, then feel: How does the breathing space feel now?

■ **Awareness of Body Regions**

Rub different parts of the body until a certain warmth is generated there and they are thus clearly felt. Then direct your breathing there. Take care of the following areas little by little:

Right arm

1. Start your strokes with the left hand, rubbing successively – the right shoulder – the right side of the neck – the right upper arm – the right lower arm – the right hand.

Left arm

2. Then do the same with the right hand on the other side of the body.

Other body regions

3. Afterwards you can rub the abdomen – the lumbar region –
   each of the right and left leg – or the head, and direct your
   breath there.

Feel the resulting warmth and relaxation on the treated regions
for about 30 seconds.

- **Hit Pain Peak**

Imagine that the inhalation has a beginning, for example, in
the form of a small ball or a small tip.

1. With each inhalation, this tip should be directed exactly to
   the point of pain – even more precisely: to the most painful
   point in the area of pain – it should hit it as precisely as
   possible.
2. Then, with each exhalation, let the tension flow out of the
   body/out of the pain site, taking a little of the pain with it.
3. Feel for yourself – what has changed?

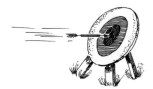

This exercise can provide tremendous relaxation and pain
reduction in that area.

- **Feel Power**

1. Become aware of how with each inhalation oxygen,   Inhale
   strength, energy, feeling of freshness are absorbed and flow
   into the body.

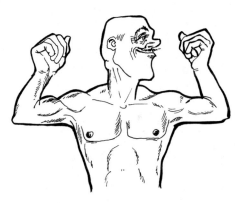

2. When you exhale, you intensely feel the distribution of oxy-
   gen/force/energy in the body and at the same time the
   release of what has been used up, what is superfluous, to
   the outside world.
3. Repeat the sequence several times and then feel: How do
   you feel now?

> Should dizziness or discomfort occur during the breathing exercise, simply switch from the breathing exercise to the usual breathing rhythm. Then continue breathing normally – and try again later.

Relaxation Through Fantasy Journeys

Figurative imagination exercises – as stand-alone exercises or as a building block of other techniques – deepen relaxation, support physiological and psychovegetative processes of the body, and strengthen positive experience. They require intensive practice, but then have a very pain-relieving effect.

Picture a beautiful situation

In the process, fantasy images or pictorial memories are presented internally and experienced as intensively as possible with all the senses. It is helpful if a relaxation method or body awareness is carried out beforehand.

You can use real experienced landscapes as a starting point, orientate yourself on guided guidelines or create your own spaces and places.

Possible theme images could be:
- Experience situation on the beach,
- Observe surroundings in the forest,
- are in a meadow,
- follow the course of the stream,
- to be carried by a boat on the water,
- look at a tree at different times of the year,
- experience a walk through the rainforest.

Choose one of the above examples and try it out.

Exercise 26: On the Beach

Experience a guided situation on the beach.

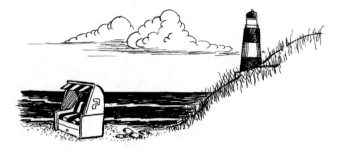

Implementation   At the beginning and end of the exercise, rate the instantaneous pain level on a scale of 0–10.

Find a suitable position, perhaps lying or sitting. Make yourself comfortable and then close your eyes [...].

Relax by using a relaxation technique that is comfortable to you [...].

Relaxation initiation

Now imagine: You are on a quiet, lonely beach. It is a warm, sunny day and you are walking along the beach [...]. You feel the warm sand between your toes [...]. You feel the pleasantly warm sun on your skin [...]. You breathe in the fresh, salty sea air [...]. You look at the sky, the colour, the drifting clouds [...]. You go to the water and wade in it. Feel the pleasantly cool water [...], the light breeze on your skin [...]. Listen to the waves breaking on the beach [...]. Sit on a rock and look far out to sea [...]. See how the light dances on the waves [...], how the surf rolls in evenly [...], hear the roar [...], and feel the calm, relaxed feeling that this sight triggers in you [...].

On a warm, sunny Beach ...

Enjoy it for a while [...].

Then gradually come back into the room here [...], loll and stretch [...] and then open your eyes [...]. You will remain fresh and relaxed ...

... you can completely relax

(From: Wagner-Link 2005)

How does it feel now in your body [...] – which value do you mark on the pain scale? You can still feel and enjoy for a while ...

Exercise 27: Waterfall

The following exercise example deals with a situation around a waterfall.

■■ Implementation

Before and after the exercise, determine the current value of your pain on the scale of 0–10.

For better success, a relaxation method, a breathing technique or body awareness can be helpful beforehand.

Relaxation initiation

After you have gone into deep relaxation at your own rhythm to feel at ease [...], you can imagine going to a warm waterfall in a warm land [...]. Pay attention once to the splashing or slightly roaring sound near the waterfall [...] And before you go there, first notice the stream that drains the water [...]. Go to the stream, dip your foot in it to find that the water is pleasantly warm [...].

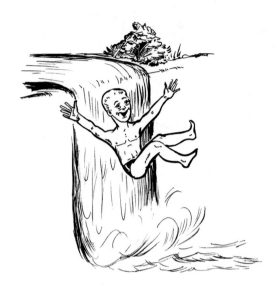

Feel the pleasant waterfall …

Then move towards the waterfall, you stand directly under it and feel how pleasantly warm the water falls on your head and massages it […], perhaps as if you were standing under the shower at home […]. Keep your mouth slightly open to get enough air – breathe out and in calmly […]. Feel not only your head but also your shoulders being massaged by the waterfall […]. Enjoy the warmth outside in the great outdoors […]. How deep are your legs in the water? Up to your knees, up to your thighs […]? Would you like to linger a little longer […]? If your body is hot, it will experience a slight cooling here – under the warm waterfall – and if your body is cold, it will receive a pleasant warmth here in which it can properly recover […].

… which relaxes and refreshes you

And perhaps pay attention to how a pleasant freshness rises from the water in which you are standing […]. It spreads a pleasant invigorating feeling, so that you become looser and lighter, relieve yourself […].

Maybe you remember how you used to have a really pleasant bath, when you felt really good and strong and relaxed at the same time […].

Lift your head once under the waterfall so that you can see clearly straight ahead and take a sip of the refreshing water […]. You will feel this freshness as it spreads through your body. Enjoy the freshness […]!

Take with you what was pleasant

Now slowly finish this exercise and say goodbye to the inner images at your own pace: you step out of the waterfall and let yourself be dried, by warm, pleasant rays of the sun […]. You take with you what you could use, the unusable has been washed away by the water […].

(From: Böckmann 2001)

Spend a moment more – and enjoy …

Self-Hypnosis: Deep Relaxation

Hypnosis procedures are among the oldest methods of psychological pain control. The term *hypnosis* has very different emotional connotations. There is something mysterious, unknown or unbelievable about it, often promoted by sensationalist presentations in the media. This kind of hypnosis is not meant here. In the medical-psychological application of (self-)hypnosis it is essentially about strengthening the intuition, the subconscious. In contrast, rational, critical, logical thinking tends to predominate in everyday consciousness.

Hypnosis as a well-tried pain control technique

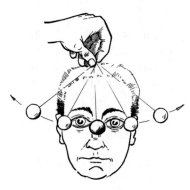

Thereby a concentrated attention is directed to a few inner processes, which are then experienced all the more intensely. Thinking and experiencing are more accessible to change in this state, but without losing control over oneself or one's thinking! It is rather the case that the brain activity calms down and one feels particularly intensely relaxed both mentally and physically – something like just before falling asleep.

Attention Focus

A hypnosis exercise is made up of various elements, these include:

The Introduction and its deepening. This is the path to deep relaxation.

Trance induction

Imaginations are inner imaginative images that appeal to as many senses as possible and allow positive remembered emotions to be experienced. This is the part where inner resources are activated and individual solution possibilities are discovered. This provides a counterbalance to the pain and problems experienced.

Figurative ideas

Posthypnotic Suggestions are thoughts or behavioral cues that are meant to follow the hypnosis in a positive way.

Intensification of the effect

Withdrawal

Exercise Termination is the phase of termination and withdrawal of deep relaxation.

The effectiveness of hypnosis in pain therapy is scientifically very well proven! The successes can actually be amazing. Within the hypnotic state it can come to freedom from pain, so that via hypnosis a real pain break can be created. For many patients, this can otherwise only be achieved with pain medication.

> ❯ Very few people do not reach the hypnotic state. The best way to achieve this is to practice relaxation intensively beforehand.

Continuous practice is necessary

Even if the self-hypnosis technique works well, continuous practice is absolutely necessary for lasting success. Initially (for 12–18 weeks) should be practiced daily 2–3 times for 20–30 min each. Later, once a day for about 10 min is sufficient – or as needed. Often patients voluntarily apply the exercises during pain attacks.

■ **General Conditions**

The environmental conditions are similar to those of relaxation.

Choose a comfortable place in an undisturbed room and find a comfortable position, usually lying down or sitting. Take your time! It is favourable to link the execution to a certain time of day (e.g. always after a meal …).

Speak the following texts either beforehand on a recording device, or remember them piecemeal and speak to yourself. Speak slowly, almost monotonously, and insert pauses […].

Exercise 28: Self-Hypnosis

Each exercise is preceded by the selection of a pain site and the assessment of the perceived pain level on a real or imaginary scale from 0–10. Each exercise is followed by a new assessment, you can then easily recognize the differences.

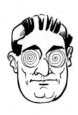

Implementation If at all possible, touch the painful area with one hand with a pressure that is comfortable for you. If this is not possible, imagine such a touch and "feel" the physical contact with the painful area.

Contact

Or, if the pain is on your back, for example, you can position your hand on the exact opposite side of your stomach.

■ Step 1: Trance Induction

The induction and deepening of the hypnotic trance can be achieved with different techniques.

Relaxation initiation

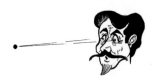

At first, concentration on an object or point is usually required. Take a target point at a distance of about 40–50 cm and look at it. The eyes soon become so tired by this fixation that they then close by themselves. If this is uncomfortable for you, then simply set your eyes to "see far".

Guide yourself into a relaxed state by choosing a relaxation method you are familiar with (e.g. Progressive Muscle Relaxation) or the following body awareness exercise:

"I perceive my body, exactly where it has contact with the support […].

How do my legs lie – where do they rest […]? Where is my pelvis […], buttocks […] and back […] – where is the spine in contact with the floor/backrest […]? Are the shoulders loose, is the belly relaxed – I feel for this […]. Where do my arms rest […]? How is the head positioned in relation to the torso […]? I trace for a while […]."

■ Step 2: Trance Deepening

In this phase, the trance achieved so far is further deepened. This is best done through a – thought or spoken aloud – request for mental relaxation and through inner images.

Deep relaxation

Choose one of the following building blocks:

1. "I am already much more relaxed and can feel the relaxation all over my body […]."
2. "I'm taking a distance from things and enjoying my time […]."
3. "I go into an even deeper relaxation by … (choose one of the four examples below and insert the one that suits you:)
   – I imagine throwing a ball in the air […] – and catching it again […], again and again […], I throw the ball higher and higher […], with each time I succeed in deepening the relaxation […];
   – I release with each exhalation […] and can relax more deeply […];
   – I imagine myself descending/ ascending a staircase […], on each step I may put down something that is currently burdening me, with each step leading deeper my relaxation also deepens […];
   – I remember a particularly congenial place, a feel-good place […].

I can also change the place in my imagination until I like it completely […]. I look around carefully, perceive it attentively with all my senses: what I see […], what I hear […], what smell or taste I sense […], how I feel now […]."

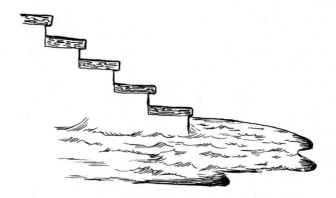

▪ Step 3: Imaginations/Suggestions

Hypnosis in the narrower sense

Hypnosis in the narrower sense begins in this phase. Concentration is now directed especially to one's own resources as well as to solution-oriented images and situations.

The imagination modules are presented separately in the later section "Modules: Imaginations/Suggestions". So use one of the mentioned module suggestions in this phase here.

▪ Step 4: Posthypnotic Order

A positively worded sentence

A posthypnotic order should have the effect that the hypnosis effects continue to have an effect in everyday life. A positively formulated sentence (an order) should remind of the hypnosis intention in the problematic situation and encourage a realistic action. Such a sentence is often linked with: "Whenever …, then …".

Like, "*Whenever* I perceive this pain in the future, I'll think of the right remedies for me."

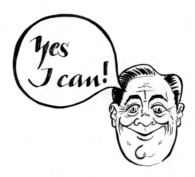

Choose one of the other examples that works for you and use it appropriately. Then think or speak the sentence aloud:

▪▪ Examples

Examples

— "Whenever I feel that pain in my back, I remember the relaxation effect and feel the calm and warmth and release."

- "I can feel what signal function my pain has. I change my inner or outer attitude and find a workable alternative action."
- "I can feel the pain gates close in the spinal cord as soon as I/my brain gives the command. I then feel this pleasant warmth."
- "I feel a cable connection from the pain site through the spinal canal to the brain where there is an on-off switch. I ask my unconscious for further constructive processing and solutions."

Try out the different ideas, and then pick the one that suits you best to work with in pain situations in the future.

> The sentence you have chosen must be right and coherent for you, it makes little sense if you feel inner resistance! Also it takes some time until it is well internalized and becomes obviously effective for you.

■ **Step 5: Exit**

This phase is about ending the hypnosis and re-entering the "real" situation. The musculature and the vegetative system must switch from relaxation back to activity, otherwise fatigue and a feeling of circulatory weakness can be the result.

Take back

If deep relaxation is performed before falling asleep, the withdrawal can of course be omitted.

One begins with the request to oneself to leave images and sensations behind and to return to this space. In doing so, the pleasant and meaningful trance experiences may be taken into everyday life.

Implementation
1. Inwardly or out loud, give yourself the prompt, "I'm going to finish this exercise, leave the images behind, and come back to this room now."
2. Then pay more attention to the sounds and the temperature of your current environment. Concentrate on the various points where the body rests on the surface and tense the muscles briefly in each case.
3. Emphasize inhalation several times – with each inhalation you become more alert!
4. Count vigorously backwards from 10 to 1 – at 1 you should be fully awake. Or imagine an imaginary staircase that you climb – and with each step you achieve more alertness and clarity.
5. You can loll around extensively afterwards to wake up pleasantly.

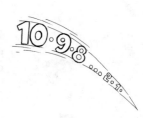

6. Wait a few minutes if you then have to work with high concentration or drive a car until the body has completely switched back to activity.

Finally, the short formula from Autogenic Training helps: "Tighten your arms, breathe deeply, open your eyes." Then open your eyes – and if you want, smile ...

> **Practical Tip**
>
> After all exercises, always evaluate the pain you currently feel on a scale of 0–10. Notice changes and document them in the pain log.

Modules: Imaginations/Suggestions

The building blocks described in the following exercises 29–33 can be used as imaginations or suggestions in step 3 of self-hypnosis (Exercise 28). Choose the variant that suits you best.

> **Practical Tip**
>
> However, the modules can also be used as your own mental exercises if, for example, there is not enough time to perform a full-length hypnosis.

Exercise 29: Pain Shape

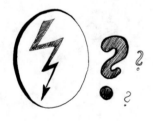

When we become aware of pain, give it a form or a name, describe it precisely, it loses its diffuse effect. We experience control over it and increase the feeling of self-efficacy.

To do this, you perceive the pain in its entire form and quality as precisely as possible and find visual, auditory, body-sensory associations from earlier experiences: What do I see – what do I hear – how does it make me feel – what does it remind me of?

With all the sensations experienced, it is best to linger for a moment (without wanting to drive them away immediately), then you can notice how the perception gradually changes.

Implementation   Rate your current pain level on the scale of 0–10.

If possible, make contact with the pain site with one hand.

"I now concentrate on the pain point I have chosen […]. I look there inwardly and try to direct my breath exactly there […], I try to hit the pain point as precisely as possible […].

Direction of Breathing

First I concentrate on the **size** and extent of the area of pain […]. If I were to draw the outline of this area with chalk on a blackboard, the following **shape** or form would result […].

Is this form clearly outlined or rather diffusely perceptible […]? What does its shape remind me of […]?

Find visual, auditory and body sensory associations

What does its surface look like […]? What material is the pain form made of, and what quality does it have […]? If I were to run my hand over it, how would it feel […]?

Can I detect a **pain-free zone** outside the outline, and exactly where does it reach […]? What is the location around the pain site […]?

I now trace whether the pain within its outline is more profound or more superficial […].

What colour could the area be […]? Is the colour the same everywhere […]?

What **temperature** would I assign to it […]? Is it the same everywhere?

Is there a **sound**, a noise, a voice or a melody that I could hear […]? Do I hear it softly – or loudly […]? Clear and distinct or unclear and diffuse […]? Where does the sound come from […]?

Is there a particular **smell** or taste associated with it […]? Do I remember something that smells or tastes like this […]?

What **mood** does that evoke in me […]?

What moods and feelings are triggered?

When I get emotionally involved in experiencing the situation, what can I feel […]? Which **feeling** crystallizes […]? Where exactly in the body do I feel this feeling? Rather in the stomach, in the chest, in the head – or where else […]? Is it associated with pressure and tension or is it associated with a lightness […]? Do I know the sensation, and if so, where from […]?

What headline, **term** or image would fit the sentiment well […]? Is this exactly the right expression […]? I let the term/image work on me for a short moment […].

What is the **most important/worst** thing about the pain/problem […]?

If it could be solved, what would it take […]? How would it feel in my body if the pain/problem was solved […]?

Identify resources and solutions

Now I step back inwardly a little and look at the pain point from a **distance**: Is there anything else that strikes me […]?

Can I experience joy or **gratitude** for this process […]?

I notice the difference from the initial intensity of pain […] and still feel something after […]."

Perceive the difference

Here you end this exercise ("Step 5: Exit" in Exercise 28) – or you continue with the following exercise.

Exercise 30: Modulation of the Shape of Pain

This exercise can follow on from the previous one or be used as a stand-alone module.

Implementation   "I perceive my instantaneous pain level on the 0–10 scale.

I am (still) deeply relaxed [...]. I now consciously change various characteristics of my pain and notice even the smallest changes. I start with the area of pain that is most important to me.

Size and extent

I increase [...], then I decrease [...] the **extent of** the pain area – what becomes more intense, what weaker [...]? What is more pleasant to me [...]?

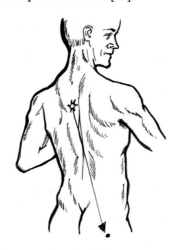

Outline and shape

I modulate the **form** once, experimenting until I like the form, until it feels good and fitting [...].

Painless zone

How far does the *pain-free zone* around the pain extend [...]? Can it be enlarged in such a way that the pain zone becomes smaller in the process [...]? How does the **outer zone** feel now [...]?

Depth, location

How might it feel if I were to bring the pain form high up to the surface/deeper into the tissue [...]? And how does it feel if the pain would be moved to a completely different location [...]? How does my pain feel in this other place [...]?

Quality and surface

What **quality** is the pain site [...], what material is it made of? Can I make the material a little softer (harder, more flexible ...) [...]? How should the surface preferably feel [...]?

Colour, temperature

What **color** [...] and what **temperature** would I be comfortable with now for the pain form [...]?

Sound, noise

If the **sound**, the noise, the melody that goes with the pain is rather unpleasant to me, do I have the possibility to "turn down" inwardly [...]? Is there perhaps a melody in the background that is pleasant to me, or a nature sound or ... [...]?

If I consciously perceive the physical signals **differently** instead of as pain: as pressure [...], as warmth [...], as pulling [...] or as ... [...] – which of these is most pleasant to me [...]?

Redirection

I now step back a little inside and ask myself:

Integration

When I look at the painting of pain from a **distance** – with everything I know about it – how does it feel as a whole [...]? What suitable expression for my momentary bodily feeling, my mood do I find [...]? If I could give this feeling a **voice**, what could I hear [...]?

Voice

What does what has been said mean for my current life [...]? Is there anything of it that I could use in my everyday life [...]?

Once again, I carefully perceive **all the** changes [...].

Which ones have done me good [...]?

Conclusion: What has changed?

How would it feel if the pain were overcome a little, the problem solved a little [...]? Here I linger for a moment, enjoying it with all my senses [...].

In the **aftermath**: How do I rate my pain level now?"

Exercise 31: Glove Anesthesia

This is an amazingly effective and therefore frequently used hypnotic standard method in pain treatment. First, a general insensitivity is produced by the suggestion of a feeling of numbness (anaesthesia) in one hand. This insensitivity is then "transferred" to the painful body part. If you complete this exercise successfully, you will have a pain-reducing effect like after a painkiller administration – some patients also use it instead.

Transmission of a numbness ...

If the pain is located in areas of the body that cannot be reached by hand, it is sufficient to place the anaesthetised hand close to it and imagine that the anaesthetic is flowing from there to the site of the pain.

... on the painful region of the body

Implementation   "I perceive my instantaneous pain level on the 0–10 scale.

I am now concentrating entirely on my chosen hand [...]. It lies completely comfortably on ... [...].

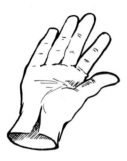

Feeling cold or numb

Numbness flows into the pain site

Posthypnotic suggestions

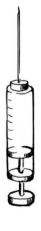

I now notice how my hand becomes increasingly numb, as if after an anaesthetic injection [...]. It is a feeling as if the hand were in a thick leather glove [...], as if it were made of wood [...] and completely numb [...], no more sensation [...]. Here and there there is still a slight tingling [...], as with a hand so cold after a long time in the snow that it can hardly be felt [...]. This insensitivity can spread from the fingertips through the fingers [...] until it reaches the wrist [...], the whole hand is immersed, completely numb [...]."

If stunning is not yet achievable, end this exercise here with the experience gained so far, and do it again later – it will become easier with each practice.

If numbness is felt, continue:

"Good, the numbness is there now, and it may get stronger [...] before the hand will touch the place where my pain is.

The hand slowly begins to detach itself from the support [...] and very slowly rises upwards [...]. It rises higher and higher, completely insensitive and numb [...]. Hand and forearm float as if on a cushion of air [...], pulled upwards higher and higher as if by balloons [...] and then float over exactly to the place where my pain is [...]. In a few moments the hand will touch this place [...].

Now it is reached [...], and at this very moment the numbness changes from the hand into ... (naming the pain site) and spreads into it [...], penetrating the tissue to the last painful cell [...]. Every other sensation has now escaped from the place of pain [...]. Only the numb feeling is still there [...].

Now the (previously selected) hand feels quite normal again, quite alive [...]. It begins to lower itself back onto the pad – and feels the same as always [...]. My ... (naming pain spot) however remains numb [...]."

Now choose one of the following posthypnotic suggestions to make the effect of the exercise last even longer:

1. "Like after a numbing shot, the numbness lasts for some time where I directed it."
2. "When I do this exercise, I succeed better and better, the numbness lasts longer each time."

You can end the exercise with a withdrawal and then an evaluation of the pain level.

What has changed?

Exercise 32: Pain Shift

Here, an attempt is made to make contact with the painful part of the body and to work on it. By shifting the pain location and its boundaries, pain control is achieved, which can have a very positive effect on self-efficacy and the experience of pain.

Implementation   This exercise can be used as a module of hypnosis or as a stand-alone mental exercise.

At the beginning, the pain level is rated on the pain scale of 0–10. If possible, keep hand contact with the pain site.

"I concentrate exactly on my chosen pain spot. There – and on the worst pain – I direct my breathing, for a few breaths [...]. *Breath control*

I perceive the exact **size** of the pain site. To what point is it limited [...]? I go around these contours several times, just as I can draw around outlines on a blackboard with a piece of chalk – and hit the exact border [...]. *Extension of the pain site*

What could cause this boundary, what would it need to loosen up a little [...], that the field of pain could first become larger [...], then smaller [...]?

I am now looking at the area **outside** the border. What does it look like [...]?

How does it feel [...]? Where exactly does it start [...]? What is the quality of this outer area [...]? How does it feel physically [...]? If I now want to enlarge the outer area, to shift the border, is that possible [...]? And with the help of which characteristics, under which conditions would I be able to reduce the pain field [...]? *Painless outdoor*

If I now want to **move** the pain site – which direction would be appropriate: a few centimetres up [...] or down [...], to the right or to the left [...]? Or should the pain be moved to a completely different part of the body (e.g. from the back to the hand) [...]? *Shifting the site of pain*

How does it feel now [...]?

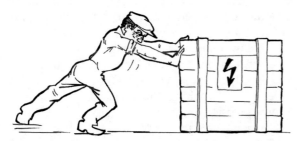

Now I look for a place in the body that feels pleasant [...]. If possible, I put one hand there, the other hand stays on my *Connection with a pleasant place*

pain place [...]: Is there a possibility of a felt **connection** to my pain field, like through a thread [...], a ray of light [...] or through ... [...]? I feel the connection and direct my attention back and forth from the pain place to the pleasant place – like a pendulum sliding back and forth about 3–5 times [...].

I sense whether my pain has changed in any way: How big is its shape now [...], what color, what temperature does it have [...]? How does it feel [...], what mood am I experiencing at this moment [...]?

I'm going to feel for a moment [...].

Conclusion: What has changed?

Following up, I ask myself, Where is my instantaneous pain level [...]?"

Now the exercise can be ended and a posthypnotic order can be connected (completion of exercise 31), then the effect usually lasts longer.

Exercise 33: Pain Intensification

Here the physical pain sensation is consciously intensified – in order to reactively achieve a weakening or resolution. You will learn how you can influence the strength of your pain symptom.

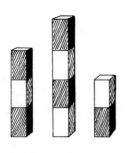

Implementation   This exercise can be used as a module of hypnosis or performed as a stand-alone mental exercise.

To begin, determine the level of pain on the 0–10 pain scale. If possible, maintain hand contact with the pain site.

Pain perception

"I now focus my attention on my pain [...], breathe a few breaths there, directly on the most painful place [...] and feel into the pain [...]. I imagine exactly what my pain looks like: its location [...], its shape [...], its texture [...], its color [...], its temperature [...], its surface [...].

How strong is my pain at this moment [...]?

Pain amplification

Now I gently try to intensify this pain: I amplify the pain sensation – I increase it on the pain scale by at least one point value [...]. How do I succeed in doing that? [...]. And, if I find it difficult, then I add an inner whining [...], self-pity [...], tension [...]. I stay in this state for some time [...].

I dare another increase – quite intensively I can drive the value up by exactly one point more [...].

Now I let go of everything slowly again [...]. I feel the difference between tension and relaxation [...].

What is my pain level now [...]?"

Pain mitigation

Most of the time there is already a reactive reduction of pain. If this is not the case, then actively follow up: "What would do good now [...] – what would it take now for the pain to decrease by one scale value [...]?"

Wait a while and then perceive the emerging body sensation as attentively as possible. Enjoy this sensation for a while …

Now the exercise can be ended and a posthypnotic order can be connected (completion of Exercise 31), the brain then learns the new association over time.

Pain Modulation Through Mental Control

Mental control – influencing bodily functions quasi by the power of thought – is today regarded as a very effective method in pain treatment. Mental modulation is used as a means of controlling otherwise unconscious physiological processes that also play a major role in the pain process (release of stress hormones, blood circulation, etc.).

Willful control

Or movements, posture and muscle tension are carried out purely mentally, i.e. in the imagination, which then actually result in an improvement in movement!

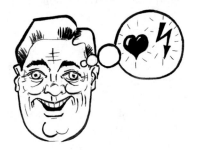

Biofeedback: I Can See the Success …

The actual biofeedback technique is one of the most efficient psychological procedures for pain reduction. However, it requires technical equipment and can only be learned under professional guidance.

Highly efficient method

However, even though biofeedback in the true sense is not a technique that can be learned on its own, it will be briefly presented here because the method is so effective. And in a modified form it can then also be used as a self-help exercise.

Biofeedback means the immediate (visual or audible) feedback on body functions that are originally autonomous and not consciously perceived. These are for example: blood circulation, muscle tension, hormone control, breathing, blood pressure and heart rhythm up to certain brain waves as an expression of brain activity. In biofeedback therapy, these biological functions are translated into optical or acoustic signals by a technical measuring apparatus. Through several exercise procedures, the user learns via willpower and imagination how to indirectly influence the signal and thus the (actually unconscious) physical processes or brain activities.

Actually unconscious body processes can be influenced

Because bodily functions change greatly under stress and pain, the practitioner can also positively influence his stress and pain reactions by controlling them!

After some training, one is able to direct one's attention inward in such a way that it is possible to control the body's reactions even without the meter. The pain is thus reduced.

As mentioned above, one must consult appropriate physicians/psychologists to learn this method.

Modulated variants that are practical for everyday use are the following two exercises:

Exercise 34: Pain Feedback

Implementation   To begin, determine the level of pain on the 0–10 pain scale. If possible, maintain hand contact with the pain site.

Imagine a normally painful movement

Think of a movement that is usually painful.

Start as relaxed as possible from a pain-free or -poor position and perform the remembered movement in slow motion (!) until the first pain appears. Pause there.

Now observe your own posture and perform a relaxation technique in this position that is comfortable for you.

Then repeat the movement from the beginning and observe how far you get this time: Have the range of motion, the amount of motion without pain, or the quality of pain changed?

Pain is followed by mindful relaxation

Always perform a relaxation technique at the onset of pain. Train for only a few minutes at the beginning, and slowly increase the time until a desired movement sequence succeeds with little pain. Once this has been found, the pain-free/low-pain movement should be repeated a few times.

Exercise 35: Mental Movement Training

If real movements cause constant pain, even if they are carried out carefully, there is the excellent possibility of carrying out the movements *completely* mentally, i.e. in one's mental imagination.

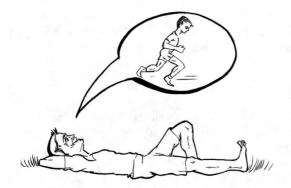

The amazing thing about this is that the brain can learn movements in the same way as real movements. Not only is painless relearning possible, there is even a measurable increase in strength and coordination in the muscles! Athletes have been using mental training for a long time to optimize their movement patterns.

Brain and muscles react to mental images

The aim of the mental movement is to activate areas of the brain that are normally activated during an experience of pain, but this time *without* causing pain and without activating the pain system.

The pain is to be trained away, so to speak. The fact that this works is explained by the fact that pain is always linked to certain experiences, such as thoughts and feelings, which are programmed into the brain. If these pathways are decoupled, i.e. movement and the associated pain experience are released, the brain can again have new, pain-free experiences. The pain system increasingly "forgets" previously painful movements.

The brain can have new experiences again

How can this uncoupling be achieved? – Through everything that is experienced as pleasant or new or interesting!

Implementation To begin, determine the level of pain on the pain scale of 0–10. If possible, maintain hand contact with the pain site.

1. Decide on a movement that usually always causes you pain. It is best to start with a light, relatively painless movement. Even and especially with permanent pain, the exercise is useful!

Movements that normally always hurt …

2. Imagine the movement you want to perform – or if the very idea triggers pain, a low-pain part of the movement. This can be very simple everyday movements: sitting, raising your arm, walking a few steps, etc.

3. Then see in your "inner eye" how, for example, your leg performs this movement. It is important that this happens very slowly, concentrated and accurately, as in a film played in slow motion.

perceive very clearly

4. Also notice the rest of the body carefully, gradually pay attention to the other parts of the body: "What is my head […], my torso […], the pelvis […], the other leg […] etc. doing?"

Practical Tip

If you do experience pain, mentally change the direction of your movement (e.g. more extension or more flexion in a joint) until the movement is more comfortable again, i.e. can be performed with fewer complaints.

From exercise to exercise, the execution will actually be easier and more painless possible. After a few days of repetition, you should also be able to perform this movement in reality with less pain – your brain has then relearned!

Different than usual

Reinforce this effect and perform the corresponding movements differently than usual:

— from an unaccustomed starting position: e.g. by movements in the supine position instead of standing,
— in a consciously positive mood: e.g. in anticipation, initiated by positive memories or after a relaxation exercise,
— in an unfamiliar environment: in the water, on the beach, on the meadow, etc.,
— with simultaneous distraction, for example by music or artistic activities, or by talking on the phone with someone perceived as pleasant, etc.,
— at a different speed than usual (e.g. slow motion),
— through other changes: Movements with eyes closed, in front of the mirror, barefoot, backwards …

Choose one of the exercise examples and try it out.

Coupling movement with joy

The more a movement is coupled with exceptional, fun and enjoyment, the more likely you are to experience the movement with less pain.

Part III: Changes in Unfavourable Behaviour

Contents

Health promotion through a balanced lifestyle

In addition to changes in inner attitudes and in the emotional sphere, it is important for pain patients to review their lifestyle and their own behaviour. A lifestyle that is as balanced as possible and a responsible approach to one's own body have a positive effect on health per se.

Behaviour influences attitude to life and pain

And just as one's own attitudes influence one's feelings and subsequently one's behavior, behavior conversely changes one's feelings, bodily sensations and mood—and thus automatically one's experience of pain.

It is important to ask: Which activities and behaviours have a favourable or unfavourable effect on the development of pain—and what should I change as a result?

Key areas of importance include:
- the own *activity level*,
- the level and quality of your *social activities*,
- Your *pain reactions* and their impact on those around you,
- your own *stress levels*, conflicts and how to deal with them.

How to Change Your Behavior Step by Step

Behavioural analysis and search for solutions

The following outlines—through observation and solution seeking—the process of potential behaviour change. Your task is then to apply this in the areas that apply to you.

■ Phase 1: Behavioural Analysis

What should I change?

If, in addition to what has already been achieved, there are areas that still need to be changed, find out: Where are there still deficits, what should you do more or less or differently? And: Which abilities or skills do you still need?

It can also be helpful to ask those around you about it—the results are often surprising!

Motivation and obstacles

If you have identified a particular behavior as problematic, inadequate, etc., a precise observation of that behavior or problematic life situation should be made prior to the change processes. So find out: When—where—how—under which circumstances exactly does the corresponding problem behavior occur? Or when and how do you find it difficult to develop or maintain desired behaviour?

Decide which activities/behaviours you (still) want to do or intensify.

Please do not forget to write down your findings– as usual with the pain protocol!

■ **Phase 2: Search of solutions**

Then collect potential solutions, even those that seem unreal- **Potential solutions**
istic at first—only then priorize a solution!

Now explore the question of how, through what or with
those who help you could best achieve your goal.

Which goals do you set for the short term, which for the **Precise target definition**
longer term? Define your goals as precisely as possible!

Then decide: Which behavior do you want to and will you
implement *now* or first?

1. Start with the most enjoyable/pain-free activities. Or
   change the behavior first where it is likely to be easiest for
   you.
2. If possible, schedule activities for the most relatively pain-
   free time of day.
3. Determine the level of your pain before and after the activity, you can then immediately perceive the difference.
4. Very important: *Before* making a planned change, analyze
   what obstacles you might face and how you plan to
   respond.

■ ■ **Examples**

— If you suffer from lack of time—ask yourself:
  – What other activity could I cut—smartphone, TV, com-
    puter, phone …?
— If pain occurs during the activity—negotiate:
  – Up to grade 5 on the pain scale I will continue the activ-
    ity, above grade 5 I can stop for that moment and try
    again an hour later (actually!).

Then get into action, try out your chosen solution. **Take action**

Practical Tip

It can be useful to review the new behaviour mentally at first,
e.g. as an imagination exercise. To do this, experience the
desired change in behaviour as if in an imaginary cinema
film—see, hear and feel as many details as possible.

When there is more certainty here, it will be time to turn
everything into reality—and to courageously overcome possible obstacles.

■ **Phase 3: Performance Review**

How successful are your new actions?

After a phase of consistent practice (e.g. after 2 or 4 weeks), it is checked how successful your new actions are or where something still needs to be improved.

Observe the results, record the impact on your well-being, and note it in your pain diary.

Do you decide to keep doing this or do goals need to be adjusted?

❯ Of course, exaggeration and unconditional perseverance are counterproductive if your goals are set too high. A healthy ambition is good, but avoid putting yourself under pressure. Stay calm, change takes time. When you reach limits, weigh up what is realistic for you. If necessary, change your goals accordingly, but don't give up on them too quickly!

Please keep in mind that your behavior usually follows quite ingrained, often lifelong patterns. Only when you see the absolute necessity—usually when the pressure of suffering is correspondingly strong—you will initiate changes. Such relearning processes require a strong motivation as well as patience with yourself and your habits.

Overcoming oneself

You know your "inner swine" better than anyone, and you know how to overcome it.

A good way is to have a reward in mind: What could you win or treat yourself to once you tackle and achieve your goal? Think in advance about three wins that are worthwhile for you!

Physical Exercise

Exercise is a must!

Physical activities are important for everyone, but for those with persistent pain, it is a must! This is often underestimated. Activate yourself physically, do sports—regularly, even and especially with pain!

Exercise or sport activities noticeably reduce pain. From a neurophysiological point of view, nerve receptors that are stimulated during exercise activities inhibit the pain-conducting system. The body's own happiness messengers are released and pain is perceived less.

This natural pain inhibiting mechanism through exercise and spor activities can be harnessed by everyone!

Exercise activities have many positive effects

— Regular exercise and physical activities have stress-reducing, mood-lifting, sleep-improving and pain-relieving effects.

— Endurance sport increases stress tolerance, stimulates blood circulation, metabolism and the removal of stress hormones, reduces risk factors and leads to a greater sense of well-being.
— Motor activity increases muscle strength and coordination and promotes better posture and body movement. One's own body perception changes: the body feels more comfortable.
— Motion patterns occupy pathways for pain transmission and pain perception in the central nervous system, the brain is specifically activated, attention is directed to the motor function. Pain is perceived less.
— The benefits of exercise activities are noticed very shortly afterwards and thus promote further motivation.
— Look for like-minded people. Sport in a group promotes social contact, which in turn is beneficial and motivating.　　　Find like-minded people
— Improvement in physical functions goes hand in hand with an improvement in resilience in everyday life and at work. This in turn has a positive influence on self-esteem.

> Almost every person with chronic pain feels much better after a year of *daily* (!) sporting (!) activity of about half an hour to three quarters of an hour. And you could say: Pain reduction is hardly possible without exercise activities!

In the spirit of behavior analysis and solution finding, you might ask yourself:　　　Behavioural analysis and solution finding
— How much exercise/sport would be good for me—how much of it do I already practice, how much do I still lack?
— Where could I integrate more movement into my everyday life?
— Which sporting activities are suitable for me and (important!) could I enjoy?
— What obstacles do I expect: Under which circumstances do I find activities easy/difficult? What could I use to get support?
— What time frame do I plan—and do I stick to it?
— Exactly what realistic goal am I aiming for—short term, long term?
— How and when exactly do I find a beginning?

Decide on a physical activity and then try it out.

■ **You Could Start Like This**
First, test your current health level: how long does it take/what　　　Step-by-step policy
distance do you have to cover before you feel a clear effort? Pulse rate or breathing rate can serve as a benchmark. You

should then deviate a little from this mark in the direction of "less"—and this is where your sporting workload begins.

After you have done this for about a week, gradually increase the time or distance every 5–7 days. The rate of increase can be in such small steps that the degree of effort does not increase noticeably for you.

■■ **Example**

Example

Your chosen goal is to walk 2 km a day. Your instantaneous health level, where you feel a pleasant effort, is 850 steps. Of that, "a little less" would be about 800 steps. So you start with 800 steps a day and maintain this workload for a few days.

If this was possible without difficulty, then increase the number by 20 or 30 steps *without* having to exert yourself much more—until you have reached your desired goal.

After a few weeks, check the success achieved and the effects on your well-being.

Do not wait until the pain has subsided

❯ **Important**

The more passive you have been in the past, the stronger your degree of overcoming will be. Just take the emerging feeling of unwillingness and start anyway.

And: Painful movements can alternatively be done virtually/mentally first (exercise 33), they still have a high effectiveness.

Important: Don't wait for the pain to completely subside before starting activity. It's the other way around: exercise reduces the pain!

Of course, too much—exaggeration as well as unconditional perseverance—is just as inappropriate as too little. However, please do not avoid activities because you initially react with increased pain perception. This is normal, as all untrained systems initially respond with protest (known, for example, from sore muscles).

Initial protest is normal

Don't be discouraged by occasional lows in between. Beware of the tendency to dramatize failures and despair! Aggravations pass after a few days or weeks, and the success of persevering is worth it in the vast majority of cases. Any uncertainties are best discussed with your treating doctor or physiotherapist. But you can do much less wrong than you might think.

The important thing is to do something at all and to approach the exercise with as much joy (!) as possible. After 6–8 weeks—or earlier—you will feel the first successes.

Sports

Particularly recommended sports for pain patients are whole-body movements in a strength-endurance range, these include: Running, hiking, Nordic walking, dancing, swimming, aqua gymnastics, cycling, gymnastics, controlled work out, trampoline jumping, etc.

In addition, gentle methods that strongly involve the body consciousness such as Yoga, the Feldenkrais method, Eurhythmics, etc. can be used. However, you can also choose other types of sports and activities, provided that there are no medical obstacles.

The most sensible approach is to combine different types of exercise during the course of the day, to practice regularly, to adjust moderate increases in exertion—and to schedule your exercise time as a fixed, important appointment!

Schedule the practice time as a fixed, important appointment

Find the right sport, do what you enjoy—and make a start!

(Re-)take Up Social Activities

Social contacts and participation in social life determine a large part of our lives. Humans are calibrated for social relationships—some more, others less. The feeling of being supported, accepted and needed by others is a deep need for us. Social activities can make us more satisfied, reduce stress and decrease pain.

Human contacts are a need for most people

This can take place on different levels and in different social networks: in the partnership, in the family, among friends and acquaintances, in professional life, in leisure time, in the neighbourhood and in voluntary work. It is important that you participate in togetherness and that there are people around you who are good for you.

Especially people who are often suffer from pain tend to withdraw from social contacts because they do not want to be a burden to anyone, because they are annoyed by their pain, because they can hardly enjoy human contacts and activities.

Pain often leads to social withdrawal

Because of this and the fear of amplified pain, many activities such as hobbies or sports are abandoned or severely restricted over time. The pain increasingly determines the rhythm of life and the radius of action.

However, studies show that withdrawal is more likely to increase pain and lead to chronification because positive reinforcers such as fun, pleasure, and real interpersonal support are removed.

Although understandable that you have little desire to socialize when in pain, get over it—to the right degree, of course—and find social activities that are enjoyable or that you would like to do (again). Building up positive social related activities acts like an antidepressant.

Building positive activities

❯ If, quite independently of pain, you react with excessive anxiety towards other people and social contacts trigger major stress reactions, you should discuss this with your doctor or therapist.

Reflect on your interests and social activities. Of course, you can include hobbies that you like to do alone (e.g. gardening, DIY), but do not avoid other people in general.

What activity would you enjoy doing?

List possible activities once and consider unusual ideas first!

Questions like these can help:

— What specifically do I feel limited in? What did I like to do in the past, which activities have I avoided recently or even given up completely?

— What arouses my interest, which activities would I really like to resume, which ones would I like to develop in the future?

— Are there reasons other than pain itself that keep me from participating in life—such as fear of pain, comfort, lost confidence, lack of social opportunities, etc.?

What do I avoid when in pain?

— Where does pain offer me a certain protection against excessive demands, where does it have a signal function? Where is this protective shield exaggerated, where does it "protect" me inappropriately or too early?

Answering these questions requires an open approach to yourself and your feelings. As a rule, we avoid things that arouse unwillingness and resistance in us. It is important to recognize these feelings and to look at them independently of the pain. And maybe you have the courage to overcome these obstacles.

Breaking the pain spiral

If pain or the fear of pain remains as the main reason for avoidance, you should decide after medical clarification which hobbies, movements and social activities are safely allowed for you. Even if it is of course not much fun if motion patters and activities are initially accompanied by increased pain—beware of the tendency to give up more and more! It would be fatal to give in to the pain by immobilizing it more and more. The pain will just not decrease in the long run. And the resulting problems can become greater than your current physical pain. Through social withdrawal, reduced opportunities for fun, declining self-confidence, etc., life becomes increasingly limited and the pain becomes more and more the focus of your life. Only you can change this!

Is a Change in Pain Behavior Necessary?

Of course, an experience of pain is always accompanied by externally visible pain reactions. Whoever is in pain expresses this—even the attempt to suppress pain still shows up...

- through facial expressions and gestures or protective postures, through restlessness or avoidance of movement,
- through linguistic expression such as moaning, swearing, complaining; conversations often revolve around the topic of pain,
- by pain-related actions such as touching the painful part of the body, taking medication, taking precautions, avoidance, going to the doctor,
- by the reactions of those around us to want to help with pain,
- by the possibility of avoiding unpleasant social contacts and obligations through pain,
- by accompanying thoughts and moods: Anxiety and fears regarding expected or existing pain result in reactions such as irritability, lack of drive or despondency.

Pain is always expressed ...

Especially non-verbal communication changes, painesome people in pain tend to express discomfort through their facial expressions (e.g. a pain-distorted face), gestures (e.g. rubbing the painful region) or body posture (e.g. relieving posture).

... e.g. through facial expressions or body posture

What initially happens spontaneously as a reflex to pain becomes chronic when relatives respond with attention, compassion or special support.

All reactions are understandable and mostly well-intentioned—and yet harmful in the long run. Unfortunately, our brain and body unconsciously experience this as a reward—the brain associates: pain and empathic treatment belong together—even if this is not your intention and you have the impression that it is different with you.

Well-intentioned—yet harmful

> Keep in mind, you do not have to deny or suppress pain in front of others. You can consciously perceive it, name it concretely in front of friends/family, and you can actively (!) ask for help and support.

Of course, this means that partners, family and friends can in turn change their behavior to support you in your pain management process. What is there to do?

Some supportive rules for relatives:

— Even if you feel the impulse to help immediately at the sight of painful behavior: Respond with restraint to relieving postures and moaning. It is better to ask specific questions and listen than to offer help immediately.

Help just as much as necessary

— It is cheaper to provide partial support than to take over all the work. Help just as much as is necessary.

— Attention, praise and encouragement should be given especially during pain-free periods, so that more pain-independent responses are strengthened.

— Avoid constantly asking how you are feeling! This tends to fix the problem.

— Don't let the pain situation take over your life. Learn to distinguish what is your own responsibility—and what is not.

Learning to withstand unpleasant feelings

— Learn to notice and endure—or work through—fears and negative expectations—even in yourself.

As a partner or relative, you may and should be aware of your own feelings, demands and limits. It is best to reveal them all. Because accusations or irritated reactions tend to lead to feelings of shame or guilt in the person affected, which in turn are answered with attack or withdrawal.

Physical activity and personal responsibility should be encouraged and supported as often as possible among those in pain. Help should only be offered when it has actually been requested.

Which Clues Might the Pain Be Trying to Give?

Attempt to restore the balance

Pain symptoms could be a valuable attempt of the body to create a new balance. If you ask yourself what the headache, for example, is trying to tell you in this situation, you may become aware of causes and factors that increase pain.

Is there too much—is there too little?

You might ask yourself: what sense does this particular pain make, does it give any clues to me?

— to a tense or straining posture—would other motion patterns, at least a posture correction or fresh air be necessary?

— on too much stress and hectic—do I need a rest or more sleep?

— on excessive consumption of harmful substances such as nicotine, coffeine, alcohol or medication?

— Very often: desires, needs of daily life that are at odds with my reality?

— Accumulated or suppressed emotions that I have not yet been able to adequately express?

- on previously neglected areas of my body or life that I should take more care of?
- on thoughts that keep circling through my head and for which I cannot find a solution? How can I put an end to them, and where are there more suitable methods for solving problems?

If you take such signals seriously and consequently change living conditions or your own behaviour, then some pain will not arise in the future.

Stress and Excessive Demands

Most pain patients can confirm that stress and constant strain are classic pain amplifiers. Conversely, pain is also a potential stress factor, because we feel burdened by the pain. This keeps a negative stress cycle going. If we succeed in controlling or managing negative stress, pain will also be reduced.

People with chronic pain often exhibit altered stress and problem coping behaviors, and most desire a more constructive approach to stress.

> Stress reduction leads to pain reduction

> ❯ If you react to stress with extreme pain, you should inform yourself about the topic of *stress management*. Stress management courses are offered, for example, by adult education centres, health insurance companies and psychologists.

■ What is Stress?

Stress is used as a synonym for a overstraining external situation, for a tense inner state of mind or for a kind of alarm reaction. Stress basically occurs when a person or his organism feels overwhelmed and his current or perceived resources, i.e. possible solutions, are not sufficient.

External stressors (such as time pressure, performance requirements, critical life events, etc.) or internal stressors (attitudes, drivers or thought patterns) can trigger overload reactions.

> Stressors are factors that we consider to be significant but not really manageable at the moment.

The experience of stress is always a physical-mental process, often activated as part of a chain reaction, which takes place at various levels:
- at the cognitive level (these are thoughts, evaluations, attitudes),
- on an emotional level (feelings—even those not consciously perceived),

— at the vegetative level (such as pulse rate, sweating, digestion),

— on a muscular and sensory level (such as sensory perception, feeling) and are all activated, often gradual chain reaction.

Stress is not negative per se

Stress does not have a negative effect per se. On the contrary, efforts, frustrations and painful experiences are part of life. They cannot and should not be avoided, because the organism grows from them. It is precisely when one can view the challenge as a valuable experience or with composure that it is experienced as enriching. The respective inner attitude decisively influences how problematic stress is experienced.

Recovery is necessary after tension

However, the body is not made for permanent stress; after phases of tension it needs a phase of recovery. While acute stress can mean a meaningful activation for the organism, chronic stress becomes an overload. This is exactly what happens with smouldering conflicts, permanent fear or helplessness. If a long-lasting alarm reaction remains in the body, it can damage the organism in the long run, both physically and mentally.

■ **Stress Management**

How can (permanent) stress now be reduced, overcome or rendered harmless?

Three approaches to stress management

There are basically three approaches to stress management—the following factors can potentially be influenced:

— *external* stressors (originating from environmental conditions, from fellow human beings, from the current situation and circumstances in which one lives),

— *internal* stressors (based on one's own thoughts, affects, personal attitudes and evaluations),

— *one's own reactions* (the body's reactions, one's own actions and behaviour in relation to experienced stress).

Practical Tip

If you want to manage stress better, start by asking yourself the following questions:

What is going well in my life, and where am I under a lot of strain?

What factors trigger or intensify stress in me?

Problem analysis strategies

You can also use the problem analysis strategies in the section "How to Change Your Behavior Step by Step" (pages 118–120).

Detecting and Changing External Stress Influences

- What areas of your life do you find stressful?
  - How satisfied are you with your private life in terms of partnership, family and circle of friends?
  - When you think about your job, what is your current level of job satisfaction?
  - In addition to good social relationships, the work environment is of enormous importance for life satisfaction; it can become a major stress factor if the relationship with colleagues, superiors, in short the working atmosphere, is not right.
  - What do you like—and what not?
  - What would you need to feel comfortable?
  - Where can you or others effect change?
  - What skills will you use to achieve your goal? And what skills would you need to learn or develop first?
- Take a look at your daily routine:
  - In which situations do you (still) get under stress: where—when—where exactly? — Everyday stress situations
  - Where and how can you simplify your work and tasks through improved planning, making them more efficient?
- Where and when are there opportunities to reduce, to postpone or involve others in stressful situations?
- Where do I need to set priorities: What is important and urgent at the same time?
- Do you take enough time to relax? — Time and leisure for recreation
- Where and when is there an opportunity to retreat and take a break? Can you allow yourself that, or does that in turn cause you stress?
- How can you plan your time better? Where can you reduce time pressure, e.g. by scheduling longer periods of time and thus creating free space for yourself?
- If two needs exist at the same time (e.g. the desire for rest and at the same time the need to study for an exam): How can they be brought together or sensibly fulfilled one after the other?

> When it comes to highly stressful areas of your life, problems that you can no longer handle on your own, don't be afraid to ask others for help.

Find opportunities for change wherever you can. There are probably more of them than you think at the first moment. Be creative, collect different solution variants and then try them out! — Finding different ways to change

Recognizing and Changing Inner Attitudes

Inner Drivers

Often it is not only environmental factors, but our own thoughts and attitudes that act like inner drivers and put the organism on alert. They are very useful in suitable situations, but if they act uncontrollably or permanently, they tend to block constructive solutions to problems. They can be recognized by inner sentences like: I absolutely must/should ... This must not be so ... I am 100% right ...

High expectations of oneself

Stress-promoting attitudes are, for example, high expectations of oneself, of others and of life. If they are not met to the extent hoped for, life is experienced as unfair and unjust. This is understandable, but makes little sense.

Fears

Other typical inner stress triggers are fears of any kind: too much fear for one's health, for close people, fear of criticism, of losing one's job, etc. Many people find it difficult to accept some of the uncertainties of life—but this makes life particularly difficult for themselves, especially when it concerns areas that they themselves cannot influence.

High performance demands on oneself as well as on others, excessive expectations and frequent inner resistance make people impatient, frustrated, make them feel guilty—and trigger stressful experiences.

Change the inner attitude

So if the stressors are in the cognitive-emotional area, in one's own evaluations and views, or if external circumstances cannot be changed any further, then one will have to change one's inner attitude towards the situation if one wants to achieve stress reduction and more serenity.

Questions like these can help:
- What inner drivers, critics, insecurities do I have?
- In what situations do they occur?
- What feelings do they trigger in me? What behavior do they lead to?
- Where could I take the pressure out, turn a "I have to/it has to be this way" into a "It would be desirable ..., it would be possible ..."?

Which inner attitudes help me?

- Which inner attitudes are useful and lead to meaningful behavior—and which ones tend to inhibit me? Which of them do I want to change (first)?

Exercises to control and change your own thought patterns, personal attitudes and evaluations can be found in Part II of this book.

Increasing Stress Resilience and Strengthening Regeneration

Not all external or internal stress factors can or should be avoided. In order not to be overwhelmed then, it makes sense to increase one's stress resistance and to conserve one's strength. What strengthens one's own resilience, how does serenity and physical-mental regeneration become possible?

Physical-mental regeneration

A strengthening of the regeneration as well as an increase of the stress resistance is possible, if you consider the following points:

- Practice and practice a relaxation technique regularly.
- Ensure regular exercise and sporting activities.
- Take regular breaks—that way you can "switch off" both physically and mentally.
- Create a balance for yourself through hobbies, leisure activities and your own interests. But do not fall into "leisure time stress" either.
- Bring the work-life balance into a sensible, workable balance.

Recreation and stress inoculation

- Seek social support and contact with friends wherever possible.
- Make sure you get enough sleep and a proper day-night-rhythm.
- Create space for yourself, strengthen your distance to stressful things by changing your perspective and inner attitudes. Of course, this also means having to detach yourself from the past …
- They relieve themselves by acting out their emotions in a controlled manner within a "protected framework"—e.g. through (imaginary) scolding, physical release in movement, feeling and allowing grief, etc.
- You can express yourself and your emotions through personal conversations, through painting, free dancing, etc.
- Learn and practice to accept and endure—or work through—internal and external stressors.

Accepting stressors

- Take the heaviness of tense situations every now and then by using humor. If you can laugh in an awkward situation, or don't take yourself and those around you so seriously -it's relaxing.
- Expose yourself to stressful situations from time to time in everyday life and meet them with changed ways of thinking and behaving (more relaxed/interested/amused). Try out the change in practice!
- Train your senses, live in the here and now through pleasure training and mindfulness (Exercises 8 and 9), this calms and lowers stress levels.

Live in the present

— Solving problems and communicating constructively (section "Successful Communication as a Component of Pain Management", page 139 ff) has a stress-reducing effect, because smoldering conflicts are chafing and lead to a loss of strength. This aspect cannot be emphasised enough. Also look at conflicts that arose in the past and—sometimes in a different form—still have an effect today!

Tips for immediate stress relief

> **Practical Tip**
>
> When it comes to immediate and efficient short-term stress relief, the following techniques are most helpful in terms of initial stress relief:
> — Exercise with physical effort
> — Breathing exercises
> — Mindfulness exercises
> — Redirection of attention
> — Thought Stop
> — ABC-Model
> — Relaxation methods

Dealing with stress more competently

So the question is not only how to avoid stress, but how to make yourself more "immune" to it. This makes you more balanced and calm, you will learn to deal with stress more competently.

Unsolved Problems and Solution Strategies

Unresolved conflicts and problems are, as mentioned, considered high stress factors and thus pain amplifiers.

The brain is programmed for problem solving and learning

Everyone has problems to overcome in their lives. This makes sense, because our brain is programmed for problem solving and learning. Even if problems are initially unpleasant and we would prefer to avoid them, there would be no development if we did not also come up against limits. Most people, however, do not see obstacles as a positive challenge and do not perceive problems until they have grown out of proportion—and are accordingly more difficult to solve. Therefore: Prevent the beginnings!

Unresolved conflicts become permanent stress

Only when the problem situation has been recognized and the problem has been named as precisely as possible can solutions be designed. In order to make behavioural patterns recognisable, one has to stop and re-experience the situation step by step: One can, as it were, as one's own observer—in an attentively accepting way—watch an inner film in slow motion. The following procedure will be helpful:

First Step: Problem Perception and Identification

- What exactly is the problem, what am I very dissatisfied with?
- What in my life should change—and what should not change?
- In which situations exactly do I notice the problem? Who is involved, what conditions play a role?
- What thoughts and feelings are triggered in me? Is there a pattern—maybe even a life pattern—that shows up?
- So how exactly do I usually respond?
- What are the consequences for me?
- Which part is due to myself and which part is due to external circumstances? What can I change, what can I not influence directly?
- What are the aftermaths and effects of the problem on other parts of my life?
- What exactly could best help me in this situation?

What am I dissatisfied with?

Who or what could help?

Step 2: Target Design and Find Solution

- Which goals, solutions or behavioural changes are possible in principle?
- If, as if by magic, the problem was solved, how would that feel? How else do I notice that something is different then?
- Which goal is currently realistically achievable and
  - what would I need to clarify/resolve or learn beforehand?
  - what obstacles do I have to expect and how can I deal with them?
  - which resources, skills and aids do I need?
  - where do I have to make concession?
  - what is my inner attitude towards it, where do I feel resistance, which of them would I have to overcome first?
- What consequences would a change in my behaviour have for me—and what consequences for those around me?
- What inner attitude makes it difficult for me to achieve change? What am I still missing so that I could change it?
- What thoughts and attitudes bring me closer to my goal?
- What solutions would other competent people I accept suggest to me?

Set concrete goals

Now rank the most viable (funniest/simplest …) solutions.

Creative solutions

Step 3: Anticipation

Mental acting in advance

Anticipation is the mental acting in advance, in the sense of practicing in the field of safety. Here it is possible to try out and modify without behaviour already having real consequences in real life—use this training field!

Pick the solution identified in step 2 that works for you and think specifically about how it could be put into action:

— How do I act when—where—with whom?
— What obstacles should I expect—and how will I overcome them? This is an important point—be honest with yourself!

Mental implementation of the solution

You can mentally watch the implementation of the solution again like a film—pay attention to your feelings. As soon as these are negatively coloured (reluctance, fears, anger, worries …), correct your "solution film". Modulate the possible result until your resistances are eliminated and you feel it really coherent.

If you have found an adequate solution—as noted, it absolutely has to feel "right"—it should be mentally played through again at the end.

Step 4: Application and Review

Implementation in real life

Now it's about implementing your strategy in real life, especially in the problem situation. This step is very important! Apply practically what you have previously thought up and played through. In the beginning, however, a light to moderately heavy problem situation is sufficient in order not to over-exert yourself.

Consciously allow yourself time

If the solution succeeded, that is, you were able to successfully cope with the problem—enjoy it!

If you have not achieved your goal, then explicitly allow yourself a time of sadness, anger and disappointment.

Then reconstruct:

— What has already worked well, and where has it still snagged—where exactly and through which circumstances/behaviours/settings?
— Which obstacles have I not sufficiently considered? Are they possibly obstacles that I should overcome because they have arisen from earlier—today no longer adequate—experiences (very often!)?
— Was the goal unrealistic, or was I trying to do too much at once?

What exactly was missing?

— Might my problem also have advantages, so that it would be a loss for me to give them up?

Here it is important to be honest with yourself and to analyze exactly.

Then find and try another alternative solution.

Changing a negative situation and possibly making a less than optimal decision (at first) is always more helpful than making *no* decision and feeling torn all the time!

Even if it seems extensive—which it undoubtedly is—persevere! Once you have had the experience of constructively solved problems, you will no longer want to do without it—and neither will those around you.

Make up your mind!

Successful Communication as a Component of Pain Management

Any relationship with one's fellow human beings is expressed through communication. Of course, this also applies to the resolution of conflicts. Many difficulties arise from a lack of, non-transparent or ineffective communication. Expressing oneself, communicating one's wishes and needs, exchanging ideas, is a profound human need.

Communication means being in contact

Successful communication requires a consensus between "heart and head". This means that the emotional and intellectual levels need to be clearly understood and expressed. The opposite can be found: in the eternal whining and nagging, in the exclusively rational action, in the reproach etc.. Such forms of communication massively promote dissatisfaction, increase stress factors and thus promote pain.

Successful communication is a very important part of pain management, because
1. some interpersonal problems can be cleared out of the way, that saves a lot of energy;
2. many people in pain tend not to express their feelings and needs openly; there is a lesson to be learned here.

Effective communication

What promotes effective communication?

One's own inner attitude of treating oneself and others with respect is the first prerequisite for successful interaction. Sufficient time, attention and the willingness to empathise with others are further important factors.

> If you repeatedly have problems with other people whose main cause lies in the area of communication, or if you have to communicate a lot in your job, it can make sense to get extra training in this area. There are opportunities to do this, for example, in courses offered by adult education centres and educational institutions.

There are some basic common characteristics of successful communication processes:

Attention and openness

Listen   Attentive listening is a very important element of an interaction. It means not speaking (in between) yourself, but also being open and ready for the other person's words, opinions and feelings.

Empathize

Empathy   This is the ability to put oneself in the other person's position, to be able to change one's perspective, so to speak, and to be empathetically prepared to follow their actions as well as their inner experience and to want to understand this.

Appreciation

Acceptance   This is the fundamental appreciation and acceptance of one's counterpart, the willingness to be able to take in what the other person is saying for a moment without immediately having to "shoot against it". It means treating the other person with respect and consideration as one would like to be treated. It does not mean giving up one's own point of view— but it does mean opening up for a correction or expansion that may be necessary.

Authenticity

Authenticity   Being authentic means being able to perceive, accept and express one's own feelings and attitudes, being open and honest with others without hurting them. Being genuine also means actually thinking what you say.

Manner

Nonverbal Elements   More important than *what* you say is *how* you say it. Tone of voice, facial expressions, gestures, posture, etc. are the best ways to express what you really mean.

Experiences and opinions are different

Accept Conflicts   Wherever people meet, there are different attitudes, experiences, opinions, that is normal. This also means that you can—without drama or thoughts of catastrophe—see problems and conflicts as part of your life. To be able to bear them and to express them as calmly as possible is an important point, because (often unnecessary) pressure is built up with the expectations on oneself and on others.

Without having to hurt the other person, one's own feelings and needs can be addressed. Openly formulated, instead of covertly and manipulatively, constructive solutions can be developed together.

If you want to solve a difficult communication issue, here's how it can work well:

Developing constructive solutions together

- Before you enter the situation, consider:
  - What is the current situation, or what exactly happened?
  - What do I want or not want?
  - And—very important—how is your counterpart likely to react?
  - Take mental notes.
- Create a space inside yourself, distance yourself from the conflict topic, or change your perspective on it (Exercise 5: Change of perspective).

Inner free space

- Go into the conversation as open-ended and friendly as possible.
- Try to engage with the positive sides of the other person and not fixate exclusively on the point of conflict.

The positive sides of the other

- You should listen well and remain as open, friendly and relaxed as possible. It opens doors if you repeatedly express that you understand your counterpart or even have an understanding for their arguments.

Comprehension

- You can express interest and ask questions, give the other person the opportunity to present his or her point of view.
- Instead of making accusations, you can rephrase them as your own wishes.

Wishes instead of reproaches

- Almost everyone does well with praise or recognition, where you mean it honestly.
- Try to formulate clearly and authentically.
- Emerging or sensed emotions should be noticed and addressed, because they usually do not disappear on their own and often lead to irritation.

The best way to do this is through so-called "I" messages:

I-messages

1. You name what you perceive, your own sensation, making no accusations: "I feel/sensed/have noticed that ..."
2. Then the effects on the situation or one's own state of mind can be shown: "This makes me feel/can't feel/has consequences for ..."
3. Then formulate your wish/expectation/request: "I would like/love/I wish ..."

Requests and wishes formulated in this way often lead to success, and conflicts are overcome. This does not mean that one always gets one's way or is proven right. But it does mean that you can stay in good contact, cooperate and reach your goal together.

Coping with uncomfortable conflict conversations is liberating, and it can be learned!

Mental test run

Before going into the real situation, you can mentally play through a test run. You can try out the situation in front of the mirror or in front of a representative (this can be a pleasant person, but also a figure or an imaginary person). After each statement, the role/perspective is changed. That is, once you play yourself, then switch to the role of the other person. Trace the effect each time. As in a film, the difficult passages are modified and repeated until fears and resistance ("on both sides") have been satisfactorily reduced. Above all, this prevents being overwhelmed by one's problems and emotions, which would make a successful exchange impossible.

Later, when you are more practiced, you no longer need the intermediate step of a trial run.

Decisive: the inner attitude

> Much more important than all conversation techniques are the inner attitudes. If you can remain reasonably calm— even and especially with emotional topics—and avoid both attacks and accusations, you will find it much easier to gain access to the other person. The other person, in turn, does not need to build up resistance, does not need to defend himself—and can remain open for his part.

Some people are natural talents when it comes to good communication, most others have to learn it with more or less learn with difficulty. But the effort is worth it, deep human relationships are inconceivable without successful communication.

Prayer as a special form of communication

A special form of communication is prayer. Here, you enter into a special dialogue. One can give thanks and pause, let off steam and cast off burdens, ask for forgiveness oneself or for being able to forgive others. The feeling of being accepted, understood and heard can have an enormously healing, pain-relieving effect.

You can pray at any time, in almost any situation. Even if you do not yet feel a deep faith in yourself, it is worthwhile to simply practice praying—and to wait trustingly.

Gratitude and forgiveness

In any case, gratitude and the ability to forgive—openly expressed or repeatedly summed up for oneself—bring about a positive attitude towards oneself as well as towards others. This opens and often leads to deep relationships with others.

Motivation: How Can the Good Results BE Maintained?

You may have approached the exercises and techniques presented here with a high level of motivation, and have already tried and applied some of them. The beginning has been made, you can already use new ways of seeing and thinking and know which alternative behaviours are good for you. You have also achieved success, you can already relieve the pain on your own.

The beginning is made

Now it is a matter of maintaining these positive results and internalizing the changes or possible solutions in such a way that they occur to you as a matter of course in everyday life. Then you would have successfully relearned!

How do you get the positive results?

Of course, this requires motivation. This is most likely to be achieved through noticeable successes or a high level of suffering. When the pain subsides, joy and motivation are initially great, but of course they also reduce the pressure of suffering—and this sometimes leads to a relapse into habitual behaviour.

Regular exercise therefore requires long-term commitment and stamina—and knowledge of possible obstacles such as internal resistance.

Perseverance and overcoming obstacles

Practicing can be a lot of fun, but it can also be hard work—especially after the first euphoria has faded away—and temporarily (!) bring feelings of discomfort. It is similar to learning to play the piano: At first, enthusiasm prevails, then motivation lows follow and it feels burdensome; however, if you persevere, sooner or later a significant step forward is taken and playing becomes easy again. Be prepared for such phases!

It is one thing to initiate changes, but it can be a challenge to internalize them permanently. It is then good to know how motivation can be maintained and which motivation traps should be avoided.

Permanent internalization

Learning is most effective, i.e. lasting, through three strategies:
1. if the tasks or results are associated with the strongest possible emotion (e.g. pleasure from freedom from pain);
2. when what is learned is repeated frequently. So to internalize positive changes, you need to apply them and practice, practice, practice …;
3. when one knows and solves one's own resistances and blockades, so that the "way becomes free" for new experiences.

Many small steps lead to the goal

New behaviors, attitudes and activities are best established gently, in small steps, within a safe framework. Adapt slowly but steadily, resist the temptation to want to do everything well immediately in a rush. That would be overtaxing, it often leads to frustration and then to giving up.

Compassion and encouragement towards oneself

Be more compassionate and encouraging towards yourself! Beware of too much perfectionism, allow yourself mistakes and insecurities once in a while. Occasional setbacks are normal and do *not* mean that all is lost. Accept them in a friendly way and then start again where things have worked well so far.

Practical Tip

Some people force their perseverance and criticize themselves harshly when they make mistakes. Try being your best friend for *a week* instead of your critic. To a best friend you give careful advice instead of harsh commands, you are compassionate instead of deprecating. For once, be appropriately lenient with yourself and your mistakes. And observe in which case you make more progress.

Turn your senses to the target

Whenever you recognize and discard bad habits, you should immediately focus your senses on the new behavior. Let yourself be drawn to your positive goal. It is much easier to move *toward* something than to try to *avoid* something undesirable!

List of positive goals

For example, compile a list of positive goals, collect arguments for them and also how possible obstacles can be overcome. Or note down from your ABC-Model of emotions which trigger (A) leads to which beliefs and evaluations (B) and thus mood and behavioural consequences (C) (Exercise 7: "Cognitive re-evaluation—the ABC-Model of emotions"). This checklist can be very helpful on days when motivation is low.

Keep in mind that new ways of thinking and behaving are initially still unfamiliar and may therefore not yet feel familiar. Don't let this irritate you; do and practice what you think is right anyway.

Defined times

Set clear times for your exercises, and take them as seriously as other appointments. Don't determine the best time for your exercises every day or wait to see when you "feel better".

Trade-as-if technology

Exactly the opposite, by *doing* you strengthen the new behaviour and your attitudes and feelings will follow. You can support this process again and again by using the "act-as-if technique": then act as if you already had less pain, were in a more positive mood or the problem had already been solved.

Pain diary

Actually notice positive changes and write them down. From your pain diary you can see which exercises, techniques and behavioural changes have done you good and brought you a step forward. Feel the success, keep this list close to you and—look into it as often as possible, especially in times of low motivation.

> **Practical Tip**
>
> Many people log their positive(!) observations for a long time, sometimes for years. It is an effective means for them against the natural tendency to fall back into old habits or to no longer perceive successes.

Also keep in mind that avoiding pain takes a lot of time. You may be surprised at how much attention, energy and space your pain symptoms have taken up in your life so far. So when you have learned to stop orienting your thoughts and actions solely around pain, it frees up energy and time. Fill this space sensibly! If gaps remain here, old patterns of behaviour will easily creep back in. Suitable are all encouraging thoughts and activities that you like to do or consider meaningful. If you keep finding excuses why you can't or won't do your exercises, look for and solve your inner resistance! Or ask yourself what positive function there is, whether the benefits of the pain/problem behavior/not having to change might outweigh them. Then you will have to decide what you want to give up.

Fill your time wisely

The regular performance of the exercises requires, as mentioned, a certain amount of perseverance. It will take some effort to direct your attention, to change your evaluations and to change your behaviour. However, you will be rewarded by less pain, more control over the pain, and greater freedom. In addition, you should reward yourself every now and then. This can be through small things or gifts such as: buying a nice book, treating yourself to a movie or massage, meeting nice people, going out to eat, etc. This is like an extra recognition for your work, and it reminds you to appreciate yourself.

Self-reward

> **Practical Tip**
>
> Sometimes immediate self-reward is not feasible. Then the weekend can be good to treat yourself to something pleasant after a busy week.

Also seek support from benevolent fellow human beings who will encourage you and give you confidence even in difficult times.

Support from other people

The very best thing would be to do the exercises in pairs (or more) and arrange fixed meetings. This is more fun for most people in the long run, you can exchange ideas and are reminded regularly. This increases the success rate—and thus the motivation.

Finally, start soon!

Whatever you decide, start the exercises soon—and feel the successes …

Even Erich Kästner observed: "There is nothing good unless you do it."

Supplementary Information

Service Section

References

Basler HD, Franz C, Kröner-Herwig B, Rehfisch HP, Seemann H (eds) (1999) Psychologische Schmerztherapie. Springer, Berlin

Becker H (1981) Konzentrative Bewegungstherapie. In: Integrationsversuch von Körperlichkeit und Handeln in den psychoanalytischen Prozess. Thieme, Stuttgart

Benesch H (2006) Klopf dich gesund. Blockaden lösen, schmerzfrei werden, 4. Aufl. Kösel, München

Bischof A, Bischof K (2003) Selbstmanagement – effektiv und effizient, 3. Aufl. Haufe, Mertingen

Bökmann M (2001) Mit den Augen eines Tigers. Eine Einführung in die Methode der Tiefenentspannung nach Milton H. Erikson, 2. Aufl. Carl-Auer-Systeme, Heidelberg

Brähler E, Stau B (2002) Handlungsfelder der psychosozialen Medizin. Hofgrefe, Göttingen

Broome A, Jellicoe H (1999) Mit dem Schmerz leben. Anleitung zur Selbsthilfe, 2. Aufl. Huber, Göttingen

Butler D, Moseley L (2005) Schmerzen verstehen. Springer, Heidelberg

Deutsches Ärzteblatt (2007) 21, Ausgabe 5/2007 B: 1332

Dobe M, Zernikow B (2009) Rote Karte für den Schmerz. Wie Kinder und ihre Eltern aus dem Teufelskreis chronischer Schmerzen ausbrechen. Carl-Auer-Systeme, Heidelberg

Dogs W (1988) Konzentrative Entspannungstherapie. Das Autogene Training, 15. Aufl. Walter Braun, Duisburg

Drexler D (2006) Das integrierte Stress-Bewältigungs-Programm ISP. Manual und Materialien für Therapie und Beratung. Klett-Cotta, Stuttgart

Eckstein B, Fröhlig B (2000) Praxishandbuch der Beratung und Psychotherapie. Eine Arbeitshilfe für den Anfang. Leben Lernen. Pfeiffer bei Klett-Cotta, Stuttgart

Faller N (2006) Atem und Bewegung. Theorie und hundert praktische Übungen. Springer, Wien New York

Feldenkrais M (1982) Bewusstheit durch Bewegung – Der aufrechte Gang, 4. Aufl. Suhrkamp Taschenbücher, Frankfurt am Main

Gawain S (1998) Stell dir vor. Kreativ visualisieren. Rowohlt, Reinbek bei Hamburg

Gendlin E (1981) Focusing. Technik der Selbsthilfe bei der Lösung persönlicher Probleme, 7. Aufl. Otto Müller, Salzburg

Gendlin E (1998) Focusing-orientierte Psychotherapie. Ein Handbuch der erlebensbezogenen Methode. Pfeiffer, München

Giesecke T et al (2006) Zentrale Schmerzverarbeitung bei chronischen Rückenschmerzen. Der Schmerz 20:411–417

Gifford L (2000) Schmerzphysiologie. In: van den Burg F (Hrsg) Angewandte Physiologie, Bd 4 – Schmerzen verstehen und beeinflussen. Thieme, Stuttgart, S 467–518

Glier B (2002) Chronischen Schmerz bewältigen. Verhaltenstherapeutische Schmerzbehandlung. Leben lernen. Pfeiffer bei Klett-Cotta, Stuttgart

Haag S (1997) NLP-Welten. Ein Handbuch. Schirner, Darmstadt

Haase H et al (1985) Lösungstherapie in der Krankengymnastik. Pflaum, München

Harms H (2009) Psychologische Schmerzbewältigung: ein pragmatisches Konzept für die Gruppenarbeit. Reinhardt, München

Hasenbring M (1999) Wenn die Seele auf die Bandscheibe drückt. RUBIN 1:43–48

Hasenbring M (2006) Kognitive Schmerzverarbeitung. Der. Schmerz 20:3–410

Hildebrandt J (2003) Göttinger Rücken-Intensiv-Programm. Das Manual. Congress compact, Berlin

Hugger A, Göbel H, Schilgen M (2006) Gesichts- und Kopfschmerzen aus interdisziplinärer Sicht. Springer, Heidelberg

Jacobs S, Bosse-Düker I (2005) Verhaltenstherapeutische Hypnose bei chronischem Schmerz. Ein Kurzprogramm zur Behandlung chronischer Schmerzen. Hogrefe, Göttingen

Kast B (2007) Wie der Bauch dem Kopf beim Denken hilft. Die Kraft der Intuition, Fischer, Frankfurt am Main

Klasen BW, Brüggert J, Hasenbring M (2006) Der Beitrag kognitiver Schmerzverarbeitung zur Depressivität bei Rückschmerzpatienten. Der Schmerz 20:398–410

Klinkenberg N (2007) Achtsamkeit in der Körperverhaltenstherapie. Ein Arbeitsbuch mit Probiersituationen aus der Jacoby/Grindler-Arbeit. Klett-Cotta, Stuttgart

Krämer J, Hasenbring M, Theodoridis T (2006) Bandscheibenbedingte Erkrankungen. Ursachen – Diagnose – Behandlung – Vorbeugung – Begutachtung. Thieme, Stuttgart

Kröner-Herwig B, Frettlöh J, Klinger R, Nilges P (Hrsg) (2007) Schmerzpsychotherapie. Grundlagen – Diagnostik – Krankheitsbilder – Behandlung, 6. Aufl. Springer, Heidelberg

Müller E (1987) Entspannungsmethoden in der Rehabilitation. Grundlagen und Anwendung der gezielten Selbstentspannung. Perimed, Erlangen

Potreck-Rose F, Jacob G (2003) Selbstzuwendung. Selbstakzeptanz. Selbstvertrauen. Psychotherapeutische Intervention zum Aufbau von Selbstwertgefühl. Klett-Cotta, Stuttgart

Reining R, Schweiger A (2006) Endlich weniger Schmerzen. Trias, Stuttgart

Rytz T (2006) Bei sich und in Kontakt. Körpertherapeutische Übungen zur Achtsamkeit im Alltag. Hans Huber\Hogrefe, Bern

Specht-Tomann M, Sander-Kiesling A (2005) Schmerz – Wie können wir damit umgehen? Walter, Düsseldorf

Stahlhacke R (1996) Ohne Schmerzen leben – Körperliche Beschwerden lindern und überwinden. Neff, Rastatt

Stenzel A (2004) Schmerzen überwinden. 30 psychologische Techniken zur Schmerzkontrolle. CIP-Medien, München

Storch M, Cantieni B, Hüther G, Tschacher W (2006) Embodiment. Die Wechselwirkung von Körper und Psyche verstehen und nutzen. Huber, Bern

Striebel W (2002) Therapie chronischer Schmerzen – Ein praktischer Leitfaden, 4. Aufl. Schattauer, Stuttgart

Strumpf B (2007) Praktische Schmerztherapie. Springer, Heidelberg

Svoboda Th (1986) Schmerzen psychologisch überwinden. Ein Selbsthilfe-Buch. Schönberger, München

Tiemann H (2005) Physiotherapie und chronischer Schmerz. Wege aus dem Irrgarten. Pflaum, Heidelberg

Wagner-Link A (2005) Verhaltenstraining zur Stressbewältigung. Arbeitsbuch für Therapeuten und Trainer, 4. Aufl. Klett-Cotta, Stuttgart

Weigel W (1996) Selbstheilung durch NLP. Ein neuer Weg zur ganzheitlichen Gesundheit. Urania, Vaterstetten

Weiser Cornell A (2001) Focusing – Der Stimme des Körpers folgen, 4. Aufl. Rowohlt, Reinbek bei Hamburg

Wieden T, Sittig HB (eds) (2005) Leitfaden Schmerztherapie. Elsevier/Urban & Fischer, München

Willson R, Branch R (2007) Kognitive Verhaltenstherapie für Dummies. Wiley-VCH, Weinheim

Zenz M (2006) Schmerz als Krankheit verstehen. Zeitschrift Physiotherapie IFK 1:12–20

Zieglgänsberger W (2007) Tut gar nicht mehr weh. Psychologie Heute 34:69–77

Printed in the United States
by Baker & Taylor Publisher Services